HOLISTIC EXPLANATION
ACTION, SPACE, INTERPRETATION

Christopher Peacocke, formerly Fellow of
All Souls College, Oxford, is now Fellow
of New College, Oxford. He has taught
philosophy at the University of
California, Berkeley and the University of
Michigan, Ann Arbor.

HOLISTIC EXPLANATION

Action, Space, Interpretation

by

Christopher Peacocke

CLARENDON PRESS · OXFORD

1979

Oxford University Press, Walton Street, Oxford OX2 6DP

OXFORD   LONDON   GLASGOW
NEW YORK   TORONTO   MELBOURNE   WELLINGTON
KUALA LUMPUR   SINGAPORE   JAKARTA   HONG KONG   TOKYO
DELHI   BOMBAY   CALCUTTA   MADRAS   KARACHI
NAIROBI   DAR ES SALAAM   CAPE TOWN

© *Christopher Peacocke* 1979

Published in the United States by Oxford University Press, New York

British Library Cataloguing in Publication Data

Peacocke, Christopher
Holistic explanation.
1. Holism
I. Title
160   B818   79-40597

ISBN 0-19-824605-6

*Printed in Great Britain by
Billing & Sons Limited, Guildford, London and Worcester*

PREFACE

My aim in this work is limited: it is to present just the core of a theory. The theory raises a number of questions immediately, such as: What is the correct form an account would take of how the concepts of a scheme of holistic explanation are acquired? What are other examples of holistic explanation? What is the relation between holistic explanation and evolutionary and genetic theory? At a more general level, if the kind of account suggested here is correct, there are natural applications of the theory to the issues of holism and indeterminacy in the theory of meaning, and to some of the several issues that fall under the label 'the realism/anti-realism dispute', and to the theory of causal modalities. I make no attempt to discuss these further questions here. My reason for presenting just the skeleton of the whole is that if this framework is faulty, it is pointless to construct the components of an account that would have to be held together by this underlying structure. On the other hand, if this underlying structure is sound, any further developments can only benefit from knowledge of how it is able to resist pressure.

Not only is the theory incomplete: it is also offered tentatively and provisionally. I have been aware at many points that I am taking a stand on an issue which others with greater competence would dispute. The general nature of the claims made here means that the whole can only be assessed and improved by many different people; and such is my excuse for presenting a theory that can hardly be in its final form.

The ideas developed in this text first occurred to me in the Spring Term at Berkeley in 1976. When Richard Wollheim asked me to give four lectures at University College, London, in early 1977, I developed the material for those occasions, and I also presented it in a seminar in Oxford in Michaelmas Term 1977.

A brief outline of certain parts of the theory of this book will appear in a paper entitled 'Holistic Explanation: Outline of a Theory', in the second volume of papers drawn from the British Thyssen Group conferences, edited by Ross Harrison and to be published by the Cambridge University Press. A more primitive and incomplete version of some of the arguments in Chapter II has appeared in a paper entitled 'Deviant Causal Chains' in volume IV of *Midwest Studies in Philosophy*, eds. P. French, H. Wettstein and T. Uehling (Minneapolis: University of Minnesota Press, 1979).

Many people have spent considerable quantities of their time in thinking through and passing on to me reactions to various parts of this material: for doing so I wish to thank Michael Barger, Simon Blackburn, Tyler Burge, David Charles, Michael Dummett, Gareth Evans, Jennifer Hornsby, Kathleen Lennon, Colin McGinn, David Pears, Stephen Schiffer, Barry Taylor, and Charles Taylor. The stimulation provided by the writings of Donald Davidson will be obvious: less obvious but no less pervasive is the influence of the writings of Peter Strawson about the role of space in our conceptual scheme. I have a special debt to John McDowell for a most helpful reply read at the Oxford Philosophical Society. My greatest debt is to the Fellows of All Souls College for electing me to a Fellowship that allowed me to carry out the work in conditions ideal for research.

C. P.

CONTENTS

INTRODUCTION   1

I   THE PARALLELS   3
1. Irreducibilities   3
2. *A Priori* Principles   11
3. Approach to a Definition   18
4. The Basis of the Holism   30
5. Relationalism   41

II   DEVIANT CAUSAL CHAINS   55
1. Some Inadequate Suggestions   56
2. Differential Explanation   63
3. Comparisons with Rival Theories   89
4. Refinements   99
5. Integration   109

III   PHYSICALISM   116
1. Realization and Physicalist Theses   116
2. Kripke's Objections   124
3. An Argument for Token Identity   134
4. Constraints on Explanation   143
5. Further Defence   153
6. Indexicality and Points of View   172

IV   INTERPRETATION   179
1. Applying a Scheme   179
2. Radical Interpretation   196
3. A Fuller Argument   204
4. Integrated Quasi-reductions   212

INDEX   217

INTRODUCTION

The philosophy of action and the philosophy of space and time may well seem to be unconnected areas. I will argue that in each of these areas we can discern a common structure of explanation that it is appropriate to call 'holistic': in question in one area is the explanation of the actions of a rational agent, and in the other the explanation of the course of a perceiver's experience of the world. The label 'holism' has been applied in the past to a great many different doctrines: to the view that evidence can confirm only a whole theory, not an individual sentence (Quine), to the view that the meaning of a sentence is to be characterized by the totality of ways that exist in the language for establishing its truth (Dummett), to certain doctrines in the biological and social sciences; and so forth. There are interesting relations between each of these doctrines and the holism about which I shall be writing; but these relations must be left for other occasions. The holism with which I shall be concerned is the holism of a certain kind of scheme of explanation.

In Chapter I, after examining some common structural signs of the holism, notably the truth of certain kinds of irreducibility principle, we will be in a position to attempt to identify what makes the schemes with which we are concerned distinctively holistic. Chapter II investigates the basis of the distinction strikingly present in both the action and the spatial schemes, the distinction between deviant and nondeviant causal chains. Chapter III, on physicalism, in effect investigates how one scheme of explanation can be embedded in another.

The interest of discerning a common structure of explanation in these two different areas is not simply one of novelty. Once we have a convincing account of the parallel structure, we can bring considerations that clearly apply in one area to bear upon proposals in the other. If, for instance, the arguments offered for a view about one area are such that when we consider their analogues in the other, clear *non sequiturs* emerge, then we have reason for being suspicious of those arguments. Chapter IV applies the parallelism in order to cast doubt upon certain conceptions of radical interpretation and decision-theoretic procedures.

It will be clear, even from these brief, optimistic announce-ments, that the considerations and arguments to be offered will be at a high level of generality. I am aware that they can scarcely be grasped without temporarily at least turning a blind eye to the many differences and – much more important – the interconnections between the fields in which explanation is holistic. My hope is that this procedure will be justified in the only way it could be, that is by its theoretical results.

I

THE PARALLELS

1. IRREDUCIBILITIES

Here are some unrefined intuitions about action and about perception. Suppose someone has a particular belief at a particular time: then there will be repercussions on what that person will do in various circumstances, both at this and at other times. But these repercussions will be present only because the person has other particular beliefs and desires. Moreover, if a person possesses a particular belief, that seems to have no consequences for his actions that are consequences independently of his desires. The same holds for desire *vis-à-vis* belief. It follows that, in so far as beliefs and desires are ascribed on the basis of the actions they have as consequences, they cannot be ascribed singly but only in whole sets.

Now consider perception. Suppose someone has a particular location at a particular time: then there will be repercussions on the courses of experience that are possible for that person, courses that correspond to various routes through the world. But these consequences are present only because places have particular properties and objects particular locations. Moreover, if a person is located at a particular place, that seems to have *no* consequences for his experience that are consequences independently of the properties of that place – of what it is like there – and independently of the properties of other places. The same holds for properties of places *vis-à-vis* location. It follows that, in so far as location and properties of places are ascribed on the basis of the experiences they produce, they cannot be ascribed singly but only in whole sets.

The aim of this chapter is to explain, sharpen, and articulate these intuitions. I will proceed first by trying to formulate clearly the difficulties that face theories that ignore the truth contained in these intuitions: later I will go on to develop a positive suggestion about a common structure of explanation in the fields of action and perception that accounts for the intuitions.

One theory, in the case of action, that ignores the intuitions is suggested by Ayer:

... this would seem to be the main characteristic of explanations ...
in terms of purpose. They serve to establish a lawlike connection
between different pieces of behaviour.[1]

The phrase 'pieces of behaviour' is not unambiguous, but what
Ayer seems to be suggesting is at least this. There are laws
stating that if an agent performs an action of such-and-such a
kind, then he will go on to perform an action of so-and-so kind;
and an explanation of an action in terms of beliefs and desires
works because there are such laws. So the general picture being
offered is that explanations in terms of belief and desire succeed
by adverting, directly or indirectly, to regularities within the
class of truths they explain, namely, truths about actual actions.

Such a view can be right only if there *is* behaviour (in the
broadest sense) characteristically associated with a belief or
with a desire. Ayer, as one might expect, writes of 'the
behaviour which constitutes [an agent's] having [a] motive':[2]
but there seems to be no such behaviour. This is true not
merely in the sense that a belief is not a simple disposition like
fragility: nor is it what Ryle called a 'many track' disposition.[3]
Ryle insisted that to believe that the ice is thin is not just to
aver stoutly to oneself and others that the ice is thin, but also
to 'keep . . . to the edge of the pond, [to] call one's children
away from the middle, [to] keep [one's] . . . eye on the life-
belts', and so forth. Every single one of these actions might be
absent (simultaneously) if the agent had different desires – if he
were sufficiently unsympathetic to children – and still had the
belief. It we mean by 'action characteristically associated with
the belief', action associated with it *whatever* the accompanying
operative desire, there will be no such characteristic actions; if
we mean by it, action associated with it when *some* desire or
other is also operative, almost all beliefs will have the same
associated actions. The same holds for desires *vis-à-vis* beliefs.
Note that we have made this point without making use of the
possibility of action failing to result from the appropriate
beliefs, desires, and intentions because of (for instance) damaged

---

[1] 'Man as a Subject for Science', reprinted in his *Metaphysics and Common Sense*
(London: Macmillan, 1969), p. 230.
[2] Ibid., p. 229.
[3] *The Concept of Mind* (London: Penguin, 1963 edition), pp. 44, 129.

efferent nerves: we are not resting on the possible inability of the agent.

The irreducibility we have just been noting can be expressed thus for the case of belief: there is no correlation between beliefs and action-types such that necessarily anyone who has a given belief performs an action of the kind correlated with that belief. (This claim will still be true if we allow 'action-types' to cover those specified by phrases like 'ϕ-ing if conditions A obtain', where A does not refer to the agent's beliefs and desires.) It is helpful to express this point formally, for it will become clear that this irreducibility is an instance of a schema found in other cases of holistic explanation. The point, then, is that, where 'g' ranges over functions from sentences of English (as specifying what is believed) to action-types:

$$\sim \exists g \ \Box \ \forall \text{ agent } x \ \forall p \text{ (believes } (x,p) \supset$$
$$x \text{ performs an action of kind } g(p)).$$

(The limitation of expressive power in the restriction to sentences of English will not damage the points in which we shall be interested.) The necessity operator is present so that the point is not affected by 'accidental' attitude/action correlations. A symmetrical condition of course holds for desire:

$$\sim \exists g \ \Box \ \forall \text{ agent } x \ \forall p \text{ (desires } (x,p) \supset$$
$$x \text{ performs an action of kind } g(p)).$$

It would of course have been sufficient for the failure of Ayer's general picture if there was irreducibility just for some belief: but in fact the irreducibility seems to hold more generally. We have here, then, a sharper statement of one of the initial intuitions about the action case.

A reductionist might reply to these criticisms that he would try to assign characteristic kinds of action not to desires and beliefs one by one, but to belief–desire pairs: it would be no objection to this that beliefs or desires singly are not invariably associated with actions of a given kind. (Strictly, he would have to take into account more than pairs, since one desire may override another.) Now it is natural to be very sceptical of whether associations of this new kind could be found that still permitted actions to be explained in terms of belief and desire; for the belief and desire together may fix one action-kind, but from where do we obtain the other action-kind that should follow, according to Ayer's alleged covering law? But there is no need to pursue that, since this second conception fails on a matter of principle. An important component of our ordinary scheme of explanation of actions is our ability, given an attribution of belief and desire, to combine that given belief with other desires and that given desire with other beliefs in a way (potentially) explanatory of the agent's actions. This feature is not reflected in this second reductive proposal, for nothing in it corresponds to a particular belief or desire. Again and again here the reductionist is bumping up against the fact that joint determination by two independently varying factors, belief and desire, is a central feature of the way actions are explained.[4]

Now let us consider some analogous reductive views about our scheme of explanation of the course of a person's perceptions, in terms of the spatial distribution of objects and features together with the person's location in the space.

The perceptual analogue of Ayer's view is the thesis that to explain the course of a person's perceptual experience by attributing location to features and objects and a series of positions in space to the experiencer, is nothing other than a way of adverting to certain regularities within the course of experience itself. This time the suggestion would be that there are laws stating that whenever an experience of one kind is enjoyed, then at some related time so will an experience of another specified kind be enjoyed. The difficulties for such a reductive view almost exactly parallel the difficulties that arose in the case of action explanation.

Given that you are located at a particular place, you should not expect any particular consequences for your experience – in particular, say, you should not anticipate an experience as of a forest – unless you believe that place is objectively thus-and-so (has a forest) at the time you are located there. In

---

[4] This second reductive proposal may in its turn be revised: it may be said that a brain state may explain a person's action, and this brain state may itself be so structured that we may find in it components that correspond separately to a belief and a desire. This would not of course fit Ayer's quoted description above: such an account would not explain by way of citing regularities amongst kinds of actions. As a suggestion in its own right it will in effect be considered in Chapter III.

general, for the individual perceiver, no particular experience is necessarily associated with his being located at a particular place, independently of suppositions about what it is like there – just as no particular action-kinds are associated with an agent's beliefs independently of his desires. (There is no play here upon the possible failure of perceptual mechanisms: proper functioning of these is assumed throughout this section.) So the point is that there is no correlation between places and experience-kinds such that necessarily anyone located at a given place has an experience of the kind correlated with that place: where 'p' is a variable over places and 'g' over functions from places to experience-kinds, we are simply saying that

$$\sim \exists g \ \Box \ \forall \ \text{perceivers} \ x \ \forall p \ (\text{at} \ (x,p) \ \supset$$
$$x \ \text{has an experience of kind} \ g(p)).$$

This condition is exactly the one we gave earlier as the source of the irreducibility of belief to action-types, when the variables are given their earlier interpretation, and 'perceivers' is replaced by 'agents', 'at' is replaced by 'believes', and 'has an experience' is replaced by 'performs an action'.

A word is needed on the legitimate kinds of specification of the correlations. Clearly the claims just made would not be true if 'the perceptible property of such-and-such kind displayed at place ξ' were a legitimate specification of a correlation. Our concern is of course with correlations that can be established without knowledge of the objective properties of places: any specification of a correlation not meeting this restriction would be of no use as an eliminative reduction. To make this restriction in no way confines experience-kinds to the phenomenal: 'experience as of the House of Commons from the South Bank' and 'experience as of a coniferous forest' are both legitimate descriptions of experience-kinds for our purposes.

Finally, to complete our quartet of irreducibility principles, we note that no experience-kind is necessarily associated for an individual perceiver with its being objectively so-and-so at a particular place, independently of where the perceiver is located. There is no correlation of pairs of properties and places with experience-kinds such that if it's objectively ϕ at place p then the perceiver has an experience of the kind correlated with ϕ and p:

$$\sim \exists g \ \Box \ \forall \text{ perceivers } x \ \forall p \ \forall \phi \ (\phi(p) \supset$$
$$x \text{ has an experience of kind } g(\phi,p)).$$

Here the correlating function g is binary, whereas it was unary in the other irreducibility principles; but if in the first irreducibility principle in the action case we have replaced 'believes (x,p)' with 'believes $(x, \text{ if he } \phi\text{'s then } p)$' we could also then replace '$g(p)$' in that same principle by the binary '$g(\phi,p)$'. The parallelism is preserved.[5]

It may help to illuminate these irreducibility principles from a different angle and also help us to draw some morals if we contrast it with an opposed view. It has been argued by Jonathan Bennett in *Kant's Analytic*[6] (section 14) that the utility of spatial concepts lies in their abbreviating powers. (According to Bennett, the utility of employing a concept depends upon its powers of abbreviation.)[7] Now these abbreviations seem to be possible only if a kind of reducibility of spatial concepts holds, a kind excluded by the truth of our irreducibility principles. Bennett does offer some reductions but these reductions are for the alleged analogues of spatial relations in a version of Strawson's auditory world (in which qualities play the role of places). Thus Bennett suggests that, where the variables range over particular token sounds, 'x is between y and z' can be defined as:

> x is heard at some time between any time at which y is heard and any time at which z is heard.

Bennett's view is that consideration of a Strawsonian auditory

---

[5] It may half-facetiously be objected that the fourth irreducibility principle will be false if there is only one place; for if the perceiver is having a perception at all (as we are supposing), it must be of the properties exhibited at the one place. But if there is only one place, there will be no explanation of a course of experience by tracing a path through an objective world. Explanation of the course of perceptions can then only be by means of a theory of regularity of qualities at the one place. It follows that the use of the concept of place is explanatorily redundant, since in that case a theory of the regularities themselves would be sufficient for explanation of the 'perceptions'.

[6] Cambridge: CUP, 1966.

[7] For some reason Bennett attributes his view of concept utility to Quine in 'Two Dogmas of Empiricism', an essay in which Quine writes of 'the dogma of reductionism' (section 5) and in which even the pragmatically motivated posits are said to be 'irreducible' (*From a Logical Point of View* (New York: Harper, 1963 edition), p. 44). (If they were reducible, why should they be *posits*?)

world does not constitute a significant restriction: for earlier in his book, at the end of section 12, he had written

A spatial auditory world, then, does not need an audible dimension. I shall find it convenient to concentrate on auditory worlds ordered by a master-sound rather than by the 'travel-based' betweenness relation which I have introduced; but everything I say will apply *mutatis mutandis* to the latter as well.

But the reducibility claim does not seem to apply to the latter as well. When the ordering of the sounds is spatial, and for simplicity (and probably for stronger reasons) the spatial ordering is, we suppose, one-dimensional, then the relation between sounds 'x is between y and z' divides into two exclusive cases, which the experiencer can distinguish empirically: that in which y is to the west of z, and that in which z is to the west of y. (Here 'west' simply labels one of the two directions in the one dimension.) But there is a difficulty of principle in reducing 'to the west of' to experiental terms that does not arise simply for 'between': what kinds of sequences of experiences the experiencer should expect if y is to the west of z as opposed to the converse is dependent upon the location of the experiencer relative to y and z – on whether he is to the west of both y and z, or between them, or they are to the west of him. Plainly three separate reductions, one for each case, do not suffice to substantiate the claim of reducibility if the only general reduction of the relation offered has to employ the concept of location in saying which one of the 'reductions' is to apply in any given instance.

There are two important morals to be drawn from this. The first is that, to substantiate a claim to reducibility of the concepts of a spatial, objective world in simple cases, it is not sufficient to argue for the reducibility of certain relations of that scheme: one must also show that *all* the distinctions that one can draw in that scheme in the simple example can be so reduced. The second moral is that the irreducibility arguments can apply even if the experiencer himself does not make judgements whose interpretation requires an ontology of places, but confines himself to sentences about the relations between things and features located at places: in this paragraph 'x', 'y', and 'z' have ranged over particular sounds, not the places they are located at or the universals they instantiate.

In fact I should add that it is not at all clear that even in such a simple example betweenness *is* reducible. The definition Bennett offered for '*x* is between *y* and *z*' was:

> *x* is heard at some time between any time at which *y* is heard and any time at which *z* is heard.

This definition is wrong if the ordering of adjacent places forms a closed circle: for in that case one could get from *y* to *z* without going via *x* even if *x* is between *y* and *z*. Indeed, Bennett later seems to notice the possibility of such an ordering;[8] if the possibility is recognized, the question arises (once again) of the interest of a reduction that is acceptable only under conditions expressed in the vocabulary to be reduced. All these complications are present before we raise another pressing question for Bennett's claims, the question of what is involved in re-identifying the same *particular* sound, something the experiencer must be able to do if he is to apply Bennett's definition of 'between'. But I will not pursue this further while simply illustrating the strength of the irreducibility principles.

I have to enter three caveats about the claims of this section. The first is that acceptance of these irreducibility principles does not commit one to the existence of absolute space: in order not to interrupt the statement of the parallelism between the action and perception cases, I will postpone discussion of this issue to the end of this chapter. The second caveat is that it is misleading to speak, as I have done, of irreducibility principles *tout court*. Reducibility is always at least a three-place notion: one concept is reducible to some set of concepts with respect to such-and-such means of reduction. Here I have suggested the irreducibility of, for instance, desire to action-types with respect to first-order apparatus and such correlating functions *g* as we considered. Nothing in this section suggests that the claims should be generalized to other means of reduction. Third, it may be suggested that, for all we know, the third irreducibility principle, of location to experience-kinds, is false: it might transpire according to our best physical theory that places have to have the properties they do, and on Kripkean grounds we might want to say they had those properties necessarily. In that case I would note that ' $\square$ ' in the irreducibility principles could be read as epistemic and not metaphysical necessity: that will be sufficient for the claims about mastery and radical interpretation I wish to make later.

2. A PRIORI PRINCIPLES

It may be tempting to argue against the first proposal we considered from Ayer thus: 'The principles linking belief, desire, and action are in some sense *a priori*: but the principles linking different kinds of action offered by the first kind of reduction would be *a posteriori*; hence such a reduction is not possible.' Underlying such an argument we have a fallacy, a sound intuition, and a puzzle. The fallacy is simply that 'It is *a priori* that ——' has a high degree of opacity, and very little is shown by failures of substitution within it. (We can hardly show that water is not H_2O on the ground that it is *a priori* that water is water, but not *a priori* that water is H_2O.) The sound intuition is that the principles linking belief, desire, and action do seem to have a different status from scientific laws. The puzzle is that they can hardly be without qualification *a priori* – for how could attribution of belief and desire then be explanatory of action?

Can we state a principle which would account for the irreducibilities, and also define the application of 'intentional' in such a way that precisely those events of ϕ-ing are intentional that are explained by singular statements in conjunction with that principle? To state such a principle would be to take the first step towards answering the questions of the last paragraph. A first shot at stating such a principle might be this:

it is *a priori* that for all ϕ, p, and x there are conditions C such that if x desires that p and believes that if he ϕ's then p, and condition C obtains, then x ϕ's.

(The conditions C are meant to capture the agent's physical and psychological ability conditions.) This is a very crude and unacceptable statement. (Above all, it ignores the role of intentions.) But before we refine it, let us look at some of its features, for they are preserved in the necessary refinements, while being more obvious in this simple statement.

Such a principle would account for our irreducibilities. If the agent desires that p, then from this principle we cannot expect any particular kind of action until we know the agent's beliefs of the form 'If I ϕ, then p.' Conversely, given knowledge of all his beliefs, we do not know which will issue in action until we know which p's he desires. (This is not to say that such a principle accounts for all of the intuitions with which we started, but that it accounts for only that part of them expressed in the irreducibility principles.)

Let us turn to some qualifications of and observations on this principle.

(i) From the admission of some refinement of this principle to a special (as yet not properly specified) status, it by no means follows that beliefs and desires are not causes of actions:[9] there is, for instance, as we shall see, an analogous principle of similar status governing the indisputably causal concept of perception. It should also be noted that an *a priori* status for the principle is not impugned by saying that the presence of the agent's desire is 'to be established independently of his taking any steps to satisfy it'.[10] That is too close to arguing that 'Tuesday comes immediately after Monday' has no special status on the ground that we may establish that it is Monday independently of its being the day before Tuesday.

(ii) A query may fairly be raised over whether the clause 'there are conditions C such that . . .' does not trivialize the principle: for plainly for any p and q at all, it is *a priori* that there is some condition C such that if p and C obtains, then q. (Just take the condition $p \supset q$ itself.) The restriction on C here needed to avoid triviality is a familiar one from the theory of scientific explanation generally. Proponents of the covering law model of explanation are naturally eager to exclude, as a legitimate explanation of Ga, that both $\forall x(Fx \supset Gx)$ and $(\sim Fa) \supset Ga$ hold, where the universal conditional is vacuously true. The restriction that has emerged[11] to avoid this is roughly that it must, as things actually are, be possible to verify the

---

[9] *Pace* Charles Taylor in *The Explanation of Behaviour* (London: Routledge, 1964), p. 33: 'I could not be said to intend *X* if, even with no obstacles or other countervening factors, I still didn't do it. *Thus* my intention is not a causal antecedent of my behaviour' (my emphasis).

[10] Ayer, 'Man as a Subject for Science', *Metaphysics and Common Sense*, p. 233.

[11] See David Kaplan, 'Explanation Revisited', *Philosophy of Science* 28 (1961): 429–36.

singular sentences of the explanans without thereby either verifying the explanandum or falsifying the remainder of the explanans. Here 'verify' means 'establish to be true by deduction from true singular atomic sentences'. Thus in the little example just given, the only way one could verify in this sense in the specified circumstances that ($\sim Fa$) $\supset Ga$ is true, would be to establish the truth of Ga, which is the explanandum. I shall take it that an analogous restriction is in force in the case of our *a priori* principle. This will exclude the case of the C obtained by conditionalizing the consequent to the remainder of the *a priori* principle, because its verification on the basis of its components would involve either the verification of 'x ϕ's intentionally' (for a given value of the variable) or the falsification of the rest of the antecedent. Since the principle is meant to play some explanatory role (of which more below) when the existential quantifier is instantiated, the rationale for this restriction in the theory of explanation accrues to its application here too.[12]

(iii) Suppose without telling him we feed a man with a drug that distorts his visual field: then we may have an example of a man who has an appropriate causal chain from his desire to drink and belief that there is a glass of water in front of him, who is physically and psychologically capable of picking it up, and who yet fails to do so – for he reaches out to the wrong place. We need this revision: the conditional in the principle we are discussing should have as consequent only that the agent

---

[12] Nothing I have written rules out the case in which the existential quantifier is verified by a tautologous condition. Ought this case to be ruled out? Certainly a world in which the '$\exists$C' condition is so trivially verified would be very different from our own. In the action case, it would be a world in which there are no physical inabilities that prevent the operation of an agent's intention. In assessing whether this, and the corresponding suggestion in the spatial case, are genuine possibilities, it is very important to note that from the description of such a world it does *not* follow that the agent's intention, or the perceiver's experience, will not be physically realized by a state lawfully connected with other states; it is consistent with the given description of the world that they be so realized. The issue of whether there must be intermediate causal states between a person's possession of an intention and his action, or between the world's being a certain way and his perception of it, is independent of whether possession of the intention or the experience is physically realized. I have not myself found any impossibilities in the absence of intermediate stages in either the action or the spatial cases. Note that, in the spatial case, it is consistent with the absence of intermediate stages that the perceiver have a body and perceptual organs: he might have a sensorily receptive plate on the outside of his body.

performs an action of the kind he believes to be a ϕ-ing in the circumstances. This need not be a token of a type that will actually *be* a ϕ-ing in the circumstances. We should take this line rather than add to the antecedent a clause stating that the agent knows how to ϕ: for that would either incorrectly restrict the scope of explanation in terms of desires and beliefs, or require a second principle. (What could it be?)

(iv) As I have written it, 'there are conditions C' precedes and has wider scope than the 'if' in our principle, and so what follows the universal quantifiers has the form $\exists C(A(C) \supset B)$, not the stronger $(\exists CA(C)) \supset B$. (The difference is that the latter is, and the former is not, incompatible with the truth of $\exists CA(C) \,\&\, \sim B$.) In fact, however, when we have imposed what appear to be the correct restrictions on the conditions C (in Chapter II), the stronger condition $(\exists CA(C)) \supset B$ will hold. Note also that the condition C that verifies the existential quantification may depend on p and on x, and of course on a temporal parameter that has been suppressed throughout.

(v) I should perhaps explicitily emphasize that the use of the word 'desire' here is not meant to beg the question in favour of one side of the dispute that exists between Hume and, for instance, the Thomas Nagel that wrote *The Possibility of Altruism*.[13] 'Desire' here is meant to include anything that Nagel would call 'motivations' or, more broadly, any kind of goal or reason for acting: it is here applied to whatever has to be added to beliefs about means and ability for intentional action to take place.[14] It is certain that 'intentional' is not ambiguous in its application to actions that are morally motivated and those that are not.

(vi) The reader has no doubt been wanting to say for some pages now that the principle must also be modified to take into account differing degrees of belief and strength of desire, and

[13] Oxford: Clarendon Press, 1970.

[14] My use of 'desire' here is thus intentionally as wide as that of 'pro-attitude' by Davidson: see 'Actions, Reasons and Causes', especially sections I and II, *Journal of Philosophy* 60 (1963): 685–700. I wish also to emphasize that it is quite compatible with my main conclusions that some particular attitude I call a desire might be reformulated as a belief in a philosophically significant way. The reason this would not be excluded is that, contrary perhaps to one's initial expectations, it is not necessary for a distinctively holistic system of explanation that there be more than *one* holistically introduced general concept in the antecedent of the *a priori* principles: see Chapter I, section 4 below.

the possibility of alternative means to a given end. However, what is really required as a psychological antecedent of intentional action is the agent's possession of an intention, and it is not at all obvious that an agent's intentions are determined just by which desires and beliefs he has together with their respective strengths. The irreducibility of intention to desire and belief alone I hope to argue for elsewhere, but will give just one example that may help to make the case plausible.

A man in a position analogous to that of Buridan's ass, with two equally attractive bowls of fruit equidistant from him, may take fruit from one of them, and act intentionally in doing so; yet it is absurd to insist that if he does so, then *either* his beliefs and desires must favour more the course of action he actually pursues, *or* he has not noticed that taking fruit from the other bowl will fulfil his goals, *or* . . . etc. He goes to the bowl he actually does because he has formed the intention of going to that one and not the other. (I agree that there will be a cause of his forming one intention rather than the other; but this cause need not be one of his reasons for forming that intention.) This suggests that the presence of the intention to ϕ should be added to the antecedent of our *a priori* principle.[15] For if we do not add it, our principle will entail that our imagined man performs tokens of two incompatible action-types; and even if we add a restriction to block application of the principle in cases in which there is more than one equally attractive means, then without a condition requiring intention the principle will still fail to cover all cases of intentional action. But now, it may further be objected, if we do so supplement the antecedent of the *a priori* principle, the belief and desire conditions may be dropped as redundant: if the background conditions about ability are met, then the intention to ϕ is sufficient for ϕ-ing.

In fact there is no dilemma here. In general we must regard

---

[15] I am thus in agreement with Harman's statement in 'Practical Reasoning' (*Review of Metaphysics* 29 (1976): 441) that 'it seems quite obvious that actions cannot be explained in terms of beliefs and desires alone; these attitudes must be translated into intentions before one can act.' What indeed could someone who holds intention to be reducible to belief and desire alone, say about the example of the two bowls of fruit? Since the desires and beliefs are symmetrical in the two cases, the agent must either have both intentions or neither. But how can he form two intentions he knows to be incompatible? If he forms neither, why is his movement intentional?

beliefs and desires as underlying intentions if we are to read a rational pattern into a man's actions, and so have reason for regarding any of the events in which he participates as actions at all. It is the desire to listen to music that unifies such diverse actions as turning a knob on a tuner or driving to a concert hall. Intention is indeed something with no apparent analogue in the perceptual scheme, but this will not undermine the parallels that are there. There are also other questions about the role of intention, such as the issue of knowledge without observation, consideration of which I will postpone in order not to obscure the fundamental common structure between the two schemes.

I am sure that other refinements besides those I have given are needed to make the *a priori* principle acceptable; what is important is that the refinements preserve the features I have noted. Let us return now to the perceptual case.

The principle in the perceptual case that corresponds to the one we have been refining in the action case is:

it is *a priori* that for all ϕ, all places p, and all perceivers x there are conditions C such that if x is located at p and it is ϕ at p and conditions C obtain, then x has an experience as of its being ϕ.

(The conditions C are meant to capture the proper functioning of the perceptual mechanism that x possesses.) Again the idea is that an adequate refinement of this principle will define the area of objective experience, in the sense that perceptions are precisely those experiences as of its being ϕ that are explained in a certain way by singular statements of location and what it is like at the place, in conjunction with the principle. Again, too, the principle and refinements of similar form will account for the irreducibilities in the perceptual case. If the perceiver is located at p, then from the principle we cannot expect any particular kind of experience until we know which properties ϕ the place has. Conversely, knowing what properties any place has will not tell us the perceiver's experience-kind until we know at which place p he is located.

It may be objected[16] that for a proper parallel I ought not to have considered early in section 2 the irreducibility of beliefs

---

[16] It was, by John McDowell.

and desires to kinds of behaviour characterized in terms of the agent's intention ('calling one's children away from the middle of the pond'), but in terms of behaviour behaviouristically characterized. For, in the first place, intentions already have contents, which in section 4 of this Chapter I will claim to be central to the holism, and, in the second place, it is on the strength of behaviour behaviouristically characterized that an interlocking set of attitudes is ascribed to an agent.

It is certainly true that the irreducibility principles for belief and desire continue to hold when the range of '*g*' in each case is taken to be the set of behavioural kinds of bodily movement. So irreducibility principles hold both *within* the action scheme and *between* concepts of the scheme and concepts of behaviour that lie outside the scheme.

Let us, for convenience, label the irreducibilities formulated in section 1 for the action case, 'irreducibilities to intentions', and let us call the irreducibilities when '*g*' is re-interpreted in the way just touched upon, 'irreducibilities to behaviour'. Now it is not true that for the purposes of the parallel I am developing the only philosophical interest lies in irreducibility to behaviour, and not in irreducibility to intentions. For part of the point of section 1 above, was that explanation by beliefs and desires is irreducible to explanations in terms of regularities within the class of what is explained by them, and, in turn, what is explained by them is behaviour described in terms of the agent's intentions, and is not behaviour non-psychologically characterized. This is entirely parallel to the spatial case, for there, too, the experience-kind whose enjoyment by the perceiver is explained by his being at a place with property ϕ, is the experience *as of its being* ϕ, and not an experience phenomenally characterized. (Indeed no principle obtained from the *a priori* principle of the spatial case by replacing 'as of its being ϕ' by a particular phenomenal description, has any chance of being generally true when we remember creatures with very different perceptual mechanisms.)

Thus the upshot seems to be that irreducibility to intentions is the relevant irreducibility, if we are concerned with the claim that the action-explanation scheme is just a convenient way of adverting to regularities in what the principles of the scheme explain. But suppose our concern is to consider ways in which someone with no grasp whatsoever of the action explanation scheme might be taught to apply the notions of belief and desire on the basis of evidence: then irreducibility to behaviour would be relevant.[17]

3. APPROACH TO A DEFINITION

We have enough of a common structure in our two cases to make it convenient to introduce some abbreviations. Where we have *a priori* principles of the kind we have been considering, let us call a sentence whose truth is explained in the appropriate way by such a principle (or a close relative of it) a *B-truth*, and let us call the irreducible concepts (predicates) essentially occurring in its *a priori* principles *E-concepts* and truths containing them *E-truths* ('*E*' for explanation). Thus the *E*-concepts of the perceptual scheme are location at a place and its being objectively ϕ at a place; those of the action scheme are belief, desire, and intention. *B*-truths are not of course necessarily identifiable solely by their vocabulary: the explanation of an action by beliefs and desires may be under a description (such as 'changing the velocity of x from v_1 to v_2') under which other schemes of explanation can explain events. With this terminology, I now turn to two unsatisfactory suggestions about what is distinctive of holistic explanation.

The first of these unsatisfactory suggestions is that holistic explanation is distinguished by the fact that any application of an *E*-concept is potentially answerable to any of the whole range of *B*-truths for the area in question. Thus the explanation that a man waved his arm in order to attract the attention of a friend may be rebutted by citing *B*-truths naturally explained

---

[17] Some remarks on my use of 'as of' may be helpful. 'x's experience is as of its being ϕ' is not equivalent to 'if he had to judge solely on the basis of this experience, x would judge it to be ϕ objectively': that condition is not necessary (he may not know what to make of a new kind of experience that is in fact perceptual), nor is it sufficient (misinterpretation is possible). A better definition would be 'x's experience is of a kind that would be produced in him then, via a nondeviant chain, given his perceptual apparatus at that time, by its being ϕ'. (See Chapter II for more on deviancy.) Note that on this definition, given the premisses that one's experiences at times t and t' (1) are perceptual, and (2) are of the same phenomenal kind, it is a *further* step to the conclusion that they are both as of the same condition ϕ; for one's internal physiology may have changed. What one's experiences are as of at t has to be worked out simultaneously with the rest of the spatial scheme.

by our man's belief that the friend is blind; and this may in its turn be overruled by other *B*-truths suggesting the man has a poor memory. But this property is not peculiar to holistic explanation. We can give an extreme example to show this, but many other cases exhibit the property. Suppose we lived in a perfectly Newtonian universe, but could directly measure only velocities, accelerations, and masses, and had no direct means for measuring force. This would not prevent us from establishing Newton's laws and postulating a physical magnitude with certain properties that is in fact force. Application of these laws would allow us to attribute forces of particular magnitudes operating at certain places; but it would clearly be true that any such ascription would be answerable to the whole range of truths statable in terms of expressions for mass, velocity, and acceleration in at least two respects. First, of course, the consequences according to the theory of this particular ascription of force must be true; but, second, this ascription has been inferred from laws to the establishment of which the whole range of truths about mass, velocity, and acceleration are potentially relevant. Perhaps there is no corresponding role for laws in the action case, but the concept of potential answerability to a whole range of explained truths clearly does apply in this physical example. In fact potential answerability of a kind of statement to a range of truths seems to amount to this: for any truth in this range there are some auxiliary hypotheses such that were they to hold, then this truth would confirm or disconfirm some statement of the kind in question. (It is because of this that a detective at the start of his investigation into a crime cannot rule out anything as possible evidence relevant to its solution.) This sort of answerability seems to be a feature of any theoretical concept in any empirical theory whatsoever: employing a phrase of Dummett's, we can label the phenomenon 'holism in respect of the evidence'.[18] It does not distinguish action explanation from physical explanation.

A second unsatisfactory suggestion is prompted by a remark of Donald Davidson's. He writes of the following explicitly as the 'holism of the mental realm':

Beliefs and desires issue in behaviour only as modified and mediated

[18] 'What is a Theory of Meaning?' p. 127 in *Mind and Language*, ed. S. Guttenplan (Oxford: Clarendon Press, 1975).

by further beliefs and desires, attitudes and attendings, without limit.[19]

This statement occurs within a discussion of definitional behaviourism: the important and familiar point here is that, for any alleged behavioural equivalent of a psychological predicate, we can, if we suppose further mental conditions to be fulfilled, think of circumstances in which the psychological predicate holds but the behavioural one does not. This applies equally in the special case of a complex predication of a belief and a desire, and has the consequence that a refined version of the explanatory principle distinctive of the action scheme of explanation must make reference in its antecedent, directly or indirectly, to *all* the agent's beliefs and desires: the antecedent may speak of there being no stronger desire, no qualifying beliefs, and so forth: and any of the infinitely many possible beliefs and desires may potentially play this qualifying role. So the natural suggestion is that what is holistic about a scheme of holistic explanation is the fact (if it is one) that a refined version of the explanatory principle it employs must make reference in its antecedent to *all* instances of application to the object in question of certain of its *E*-concepts. This would indeed be a natural sense for the word 'holism', because any scheme to which it applied could of necessity not be a partial theory of the *E*-concepts: for one would not, as indeed one does not in the case of action, have any assurance that a consequence could be drawn from, be explained by, the theory in advance of a degree of confidence that all the relevant instances had been ascertained of application of the *E*-concepts to the object in question. In the case of action explanation this is a genuine and important phenomenon, and in cases in which it is present it is natural to speak of holism of explanation by the *E*-truths at a given time.

The phenomenon is, however, simply not present in the perceptual case. It is true that what it is like at places other than p can affect what it is like at p, but no reference to what it is like elsewhere is needed in the antecedent of the (existentially quantified) *a priori* principle that explains the nature of the perceiver's experience. What is happening elsewhere may

[19] 'Mental Events' in *Experience and Theory*, ed. L. Foster and J. Swanson (London: Duckworth, 1970), p. 92.

also affect whether the conditions C obtain, but again this is irrelevant: the conditions C were held constant in the description of the pertinent property of the action explanation case.[20] We could accept this property as distinctive of the kind of holistic explanation in which we are interested only at the cost of abandoning any uniform, general explanation of the many common features – some noted already and some to come later – of the spatial and the action cases.

It should be noted, too, that even if either of these two inadequate accounts were extensionally adequate, they would still have to be shown to meet a further condition: some account would have to be given of how exactly the favoured feature produces the distinctive aspects of holistic explanation already described. The two unsatisfactory suggestions seem to be at the wrong level of generality, the first too high and the second too low, to do that.

A very natural suggestion at this point is that it is in fact the very presence of *a priori* principles of the kind cited that is characteristic of holistic explanation. I shall argue that this is indeed a necessary feature, and later try to say what more is needed to fill it out into a property also sufficient for a holistic scheme of explanation. In more detail, the natural suggestion is that any holistic scheme has some associated *a priori* principles, the E-concepts of which are applied in such a way as to make those very principles always come out true; in particular, it is a requirement for *mastery* of those E-concepts that they be applied in such a way that these schemata (principles) hold. If this is correct, it is a first point in vital and vivid contrast with much explanation in the physical sciences. For however strong the case for saying that natural physical laws are necessary – and in the light of plausible theories of natural kind terms it seems very strong – it cannot be maintained that a grasp of any of those laws is needed for mastery of the predicates

[20] It may be asked why we do not have an analogue of the phenomenon in question in the action case, in the possibility that one quality instantiated at a place may be sufficiently powerful to drown any trace of others, in the experience of someone at that place, even though those others are equally instantiated at that place. But this is not an instance of the parallel we are considering, in which (roughly) the comparison is between the desire that p, and location at place p, and the belief that if one ϕ's then p, and its being ϕ at place p. Nothing stands to location quite as degrees of strength stand to desire.

they contain: ignorance that ingestion of barbiturates together with alcohol leads to death does not cast any doubt on a man's ability to apply competently 'barbiturate' and 'alcohol'. (It is maintained under this suggestion only that the requirement that the principles be true is *an* element involved in mastery of the *E*-concepts, and not necessarily the whole truth about such mastery.)[21]

The very fact that the explanatory principles are in some sense knowable in advance of any particular experience, that is, are *a priori* in the usual sense, is evidence for this view; but it cannot be conclusive, because in its usual sense that means that the *E*-concepts *can* be known in advance to apply to a creature's actions or a course of experience if that kind of scheme applies at all, whereas the present suggestion is that the *E*-concepts *must* be applied in accordance with these principles. To establish this stronger claim, one needs to show any other basis of application is defective. Plainly this cannot be shown conclusively, but one can have strong evidence for it if each alternative basis that is proposed is not only inadequate, but its inadequacy can be related to its lack of answerability to the truth of the *a priori* principles. I will argue that this last condition does indeed hold. In saying that it does one is not of course excluding the possibility of indirect evidence for the application of *E*-concepts, supplied by testimony or by the truth of some general nonconstitutive theory employing those concepts: one is requiring only that the indirect evidence rests ultimately on the application of the *E*-concepts in accordance with the *a priori* principles.[22]

We can see the plausibility of the position in the case of action by considering one or two alternative bases of attribution

[21] One reason for saying these *a priori* principles do not give the whole account is that they do not even explain the ideal of consistency of beliefs. There seems to be nothing to stop two obviously inconsistent beliefs both being explanatory of action by these principles. For more on this, see section 4.

[22] I hope it is clear that, despite my use of the label '*a priori*', there need not be anything non-Quinean in the special status I attribute to the principles in question: for the special status turns on considerations about when we will say that a person has mastery of a given concept. The status of the claims I am making may be said to be the same as those (right or wrong) that Quine makes in *Word and Object* (Cambridge, Mass.: MIT Press, 1960) and *The Roots of Reference* (La Salle, Ill.: Open Court, 1974) about what is required for mastery of 'apple' as an expression of divided reference as opposed to a mass term, etc. 'Constitutively true' might be better than '*a priori*'.

for the E-concepts. We have already seen that no purely behavioural basis (even in the broadest sense of 'behavioural') can supply by translation a basis for attribution of beliefs and desires; and this we saw was connected with the truth of the *a priori* principles. Could a man then in principle apply the E-concepts by means of systematic and intricate knowledge of a creature's brain states? It would be a very bad objection to this to say that the ordinary speaker has no such knowledge available. For, first, this would not show that the criterion diverged in any way from the application determined in accordance with the *a priori* principles, and this application could be quite enough for explanatory purposes; and second, it is clear on the ordinary concept of belief that what is believed can depend on quite recherché facts about the brain. What is believed may depend upon what is remembered, and whether one rather than another occasion is what is remembered may depend upon whether the contents of one rather than another information storage device in a creature's brain were destroyed in the past. The objection to such a basis for mastery is rather that a man in possession of it could not reliably go on to apply the concept in new cases. Our ordinary concepts of belief and desire may be applied to any organism that is systematically interpretable as having propositional attitudes, regardless of its internal structure and chemical composition. Quite different brain states in another species of creature or in another particular creature may correspond to the same belief or desire; without knowledge of the principle connecting belief, desire, intention, and action (and knowledge that the principle is to hold quite generally), our man could not know which way to move in the new case.

This is a strong claim because it involves saying that *one* kind of higher-order physical definition is not possible for beliefs and desires.[23] These kinds of definition are those that make reference to some particular physically specified state or kind of event; and the reason for saying they are not possible for beliefs and desires rests again upon the irreducibility principles of section 1 above. It is plausible that we can give such a higher-order

---

[23] The more general possibility of this kind of higher-order definition is noted by Hilary Putnam, 'On Properties', repr. in *Mathematics, Matter and Method* (Cambridge: CUP, 1975), Philosophical Papers, vol. I.

definition of 'valve', a definition that does not require anything falling under it to have a particular physico-chemical constitution, because we can physically specify its role of allowing only a one-way flow of a material. But beliefs (desires) have no distinctive causal role independently of suppositions about what desires (beliefs) the agent has: we do not have the foundation stone needed to build a physical definition of this kind. (Higher-order physical definitions of a rather different kind and which take into account simultaneous determination by beliefs and desires are evidently not excluded by these considerations: see Chapter III, section 6.)

A quite different basis for application of the E-concepts in the case of action might be said to be provided by the agent's own (in general) immediate noninferential reports of his beliefs and desires. Now in fact it is clear that this 'basis' is overruled when ascriptions thus based conflict with the preservation of the a priori principles: the man who discovers that his inclination to give to a certain charitable cause disappears on being told that he will not be publicized as having done so, learns that he did not have a desire simply to help the starving. Such observations, however, do not remove all of the perplexities generated by the view of holistic explanation being considered. For on the view being presented, possessing a certain belief or desire one has a certain (as it were) *causal* power in the presence of other desires or beliefs; how can there be noninferential knowledge of states that necessarily have such consequences? Thus Charles Taylor once wrote:

Our present scheme requires that we sometimes be able to identify our desires directly, that what we or others want should sometimes, indeed normally, be an open fact. The phenomena by which we identify them must be transparent, as it were, so that the desire can be read through them directly, without having to decode signs according to some correlations established in experience.[24]

Certainly a man can knowledgeably ascribe desires and beliefs to himself without any thought on his part of their potential role in the explanation of his own actions.

It would not be satisfactory to reply to this objection by

---

[24] *The Explanation of Behaviour*, p. 50.

saying that a man does not need to know the *a priori* principle in order to self-ascribe desires and beliefs, but he does need to know it in order to ascribe beliefs and desires to others. If this were the best answer we could give, it is hard to see how one could answer the charge that by this account, 'desires' and 'believes' are both ambiguous: for we have been given an account of their application that allows two different criteria as sufficient for them to apply, with (as yet) no connection stated between them. Such an objection will always arise for any account that attempts to specify the meaning of a word by giving a list of criteria for its application, a list the items on which are not unified by some overarching single principle. But in fact we do not need to answer the objection from the case of the imagined self-ascriber of beliefs and desires in a way that would destroy the unity of the concept. We can admit the case but appeal to a causal theory of knowledge.

Normally when one ascribes a desire to oneself one knows of one's desire noninferentially. One's belief that one has that desire is caused by the existence of the desire; and the desire is also the ground of the causal power that is operative in future circumstances when the desire is engaged. It is a case of a common cause leading to knowledge. In this respect it may be compared with the knowledge that even a locally anaesthetized man may have of the position of his limbs without perceiving them: if his efferent nerves are still working, his belief that his limbs are in a certain position and their being so have a common cause. The possibility of noninferential knowledge of the applicability of an *E*-concept does not provide an objection to the claim that the extension of the *E*-concepts is partially determined by the *a priori* principle.

The reply just given is an example of a more generally applicable strategy. Suppose a view is put forward that a certain concept has to be applied in accordance with a certain principle. Then it is never by itself a sufficient objection to such a view that a person can apply the concept, and indeed know truths expressed using it, without ever having thought of the principle. For it could be that the person has noninferential knowledge of when the concept applies, and he will have it if the mechanism that produces his uninferred beliefs is appropriately sensitive to what *would* be the extension of the concept when consciously applied in accordance with the suggested principle.

It may, however, be said that there is a second sense, so far neglected in this discussion, in which what the agent says takes precedence over his other actions in the ascription to him of beliefs. In this second sense, if there is a conflict between the evidence from nonlinguistic actions and the evidence from what the agent says (with respect to one and the same time), then the evidence from saying overrides the evidence from other actions. Such a claim need not be the definitional point that *sincere* sayings override: the point may rather be that if, simultaneously, the sayings point one way and nonlinguistic actions point in the other on the question of whether the agent believes that p, and we have no reason to believe the agent deceptive in either his actions or his sayings, then we take the direction indicated by his sayings.

Is this suggestion true? There certainly exist examples like the following. A person has a fear of taking off in planes, and accordingly always travels by land or sea: and this though he protests that he accepts without reservation the aerodynamic principles that entail that when the aircraft reaches a certain speed, it must leave the ground, and is prepared to bet at the same odds as the rest of us that particular aircraft will succeed in leaving the ground. In such cases the evidence from travelling habits is overridden. But examples like that cannot show the primacy of saying for ascription of belief, since it is equally possible that an action of saying something is inhibited by an irrational fear, by such causes as having had an upbringing in which such things were not said nor mentioned. If that were so, and a man's actions conformed with what we would expect if he had the belief (given his other attitudes), then the evidence from nonlinguistic actions might override his failure to be prepared to assert what we will hold him to believe. We will demand an explanation of the man's failure to say what he believes: but equally we will want some explanation of the fear of flying that is preventing a person's other desires and beliefs from operating.[25]

---

[25] Two more general remarks are in order here. (a) The interpretation of a person's words is answerable to the goal of rationalizing all of his or her intentional behaviour, both linguistic and nonlinguistic. This makes it difficult for there to

In the spatial case it is extraordinarily difficult even to begin to imagine how one might apply the E-concepts independently of acceptance of the *a priori* principle. We have again already seen how one kind of reductive basis cannot be supplied. It is true that in some cases the *a priori* principle may need amendment for trivial reasons: we could, for instance, imagine someone brought up from birth with his optic nerve linked causally to a perceptual device five miles away, which moves systematically as he moves. Then we might make sense of this person being visually located where (most of) his body isn't. But plainly such examples cannot cast doubt on the principle relativized to a sense modality M:

> If x is M-located at p, it is ϕ at p, ϕ is M-detectable, and C obtains, then x experiences ϕ (in M).

Indeed it would be noted that it is actually incoherent to suggest that one's M-location could be established via some other sensory modality M' without use of the corresponding principle. Suppose one's tactile location bears a certain relation R to one's visual location. One might establish this from the fact that a certain region of space bearing R to one's current visual location has a configuration of spherical objects which one can currently touch. But of course this does not avoid use of the *a priori* principle relativized to sense modality M: on the contrary it presupposes the truth of the principle, for otherwise one would not expect to touch the configuration of spherical objects in these circumstances.

It is of course not to be denied that our experience of space might conceivably have been of such a kind that, as things in fact were, one could tell one's location at a glance. Thus we may imagine the surface of a sphere varying in colour so that

---

be a completely general dissociation of the action and saying bases of ascription of beliefs: for any interpretation scheme that produced such dissociation would be suspect for just that reason. (b) The thesis of the primacy of saying in ascriptions of attitude is perhaps more plausible for belief than for desire. But if there is a case to be made here, it must be made on more than appeal just to differences between belief and desire in respect of the agent's sayings. For there could conceivably be a linguistic mood that stands to desire as the indicative stands to belief (the imperative seems not to be it because of the special role of the addressee). An argument to establish asymmetry between belief and desire must show that facts analogous to those relating belief and saying do not relate desire and utterances of sentences in that possible mood.

every pair of distinct regions is of discriminably (and memorably) distinct shades; the movement of small objects on the surface of the sphere neither obscures nor alters the background colour. In such a world, could not someone acquire exhaustive mastery of the notion 'where I am located' in purely qualitative terms? It seems obvious that he could not: we may press the question of whether it is intelligible on the alleged notion of place thus introduced that a place should alter in background colour (perhaps to a colour occurring elsewhere on the sphere), evidence for this being given by the experiences obtained on different paths of travel. If it is not intelligible, it is no genuine concept of place that he has; if it is intelligible, it follows that mastery of his concept is not after all specifiable in purely qualitative terms.

As before, one can only examine alleged counterexamples, and argue that they do not really show that mastery of the E-concepts is attainable independently of the *a priori* principle: but also as before, it does seem that the failure in the alleged counterexamples is systematically related to their neglect of the principle.

I said earlier that the presence of *a priori* principles of the kind described is only necessary and not sufficient for a scheme of holistic explanation. This can be seen by reference to functional or quasi-functional statements about objects. Corresponding to the earlier *a priori* statements we can say that it is *a priori* that there are conditions C such that if object x has the functional end of placing or keeping object y in state G, and x's ϕ-ing is necessary and sufficient for y's being in state G, and C obtains, then x ϕ's. (Here x might be a thermostat, y a room, and G the state of being at 70°F.) For x to have the functional end of y's being G, it is plainly not sufficient that such a conditional be true, for otherwise we would have, for instance, a true functional statement about any system that happened to be in a stable equilibrium within certain limits: so the tendency of water that is distilled in a basin to return to the horizontal would wrongly be included.[26] But the conditional

---

[26] This counterexample would not though cast doubt on an analysis making use of the condition that for any ϕ in a certain range, when C obtains x ϕ's because ϕ-ing then leads to y's being G. It might be said that the water counterexample shows simply that we cannot analyse this 'because' in terms of the truth of a principle of a certain form.

seems clearly to be necessary, and that is enough for the objection to arise.

We cannot avoid the problem by saying that though the principle is in some sense *a priori*, it does not contain the characteristic kind of *E*-concepts that cannot be applied independently of it: for the notion of a function here seems to be just such a concept. For any particular functional end *G* we consider, there are infinitely many distinct possible physico-chemical mechanisms that may operate to ensure the end *G* is attained in a variety of circumstances (with condition C obtaining); and if this is so, we cannot expect to come up with a general reductive first-order definition of possession of functional end *G*. It is true that for any particular *x*, *y*, and *G* we may manage to state a complete physical account that is of exactly the same (or greater) predictive power as the functional account: in the case of the thermostat operated by a bimetallic strip, this would involve a nonfunctional account of how the different coefficients of expansion of the two metals composing the strip operate to close or break the circuit at different temperatures. But it would be dogmatic to deny that for a particular creature with respect to a particular belief/desire pair one could explain in neurophysiological terms the particular bodily movement that is the particular action they explain. The fact that the action may be intentional under a description that is plausibly not reducible to open sentences of physics (or even biology) (e.g., 'the drawing up of a will') is here an irrelevance: first, because as we noted actions are not always intentional under descriptions of that kind, and second, because some functions a system may have, for instance that of controlling the traffic, seem not to be so reducible. In any case there are functional cases where in a particular instance the non-functional account would be as complex and as distant from us in our present state of knowledge as such an explanation of a particular action: one thinks, for instance, of our knowledge of the general functions of DNA combined with our ignorance of how it achieves them.

These examples of functional ends are clearly somewhat heterogeneous, but even if they split up into different kinds, the possibility of a case of any one kind, combined with a conviction that the spatial and action schemes of explanation are holistic in some stronger sense, shows that some aspect of holistic explanation remains to be captured: the presence of a certain kind of *a priori* principle is not by itself sufficient.

4. THE BASIS OF THE HOLISM

Let us restate our original intuitions about what makes the action and spatial schemes holistic. When we ascribe a desire, say, to someone, then if accepted this ascription has repercussions for what we would expect him to do in various circumstances; but it has these particular repercussions only because we ascribe other particular beliefs and desires to the person. Similarly, when we ascribe a location, say, to someone, then if this ascription is true there will be repercussions for what courses of experience are empirically possible for him, courses that correspond to the various routes he may take through the world; but again, these particular repercussions are present only because we ascribe particular properties to particular places. Now in considering this as the basis of the holism we need to be careful about the kinds of repercussions in question.

The source of the repercussions in which we are interested does not lie in the fact that in the *a priori* principles of each scheme, for one of the conjuncts of the antecedent containing an *E*-concept, there are many instances of another conjunct which together with the given one help to form an instance of that *a priori* principle. This multiplicity is certainly a feature of each scheme. In the action case, for the desire that *p*, there are many beliefs (all those of the form that if he ϕ's then *p*) that may combine with that desire in accordance with the principle, even on its crudest formulation; in the spatial case, if the experiencer is located at a given place *p*, then there are many qualities ϕ that may be instantiated at *p*, and which may produce an experience in accordance with the *a priori* principle. But once again this multiplicity is not something confined to examples that intuitively we want to call holistic. Consider an *a priori* principle of a now familiar kind linking *valve* with *valve-lifter, valve-strengthener, valve-filter* . . .

We have so far ignored the role of time. The missing element in the account of what makes the two schemes holistic is the *a priori* restriction they both contain upon how temporally successive sequences of B-truths may be explained within each scheme. It is not surprising that so far we have failed to capture this in the *a priori* principles of the schemes we have already considered, for all these principles concerned explanation of a B-truth at a given time: they impose no restrictions upon the application of the E-concepts at different times. And holism of the explanation by E-truths *at a given time* wears this limitation on its face.

In the case of action, restrictions on the application of the E-concepts at different times are determined by the general idea of rationality. A pattern of beliefs and derived desires over time must be responsive in intelligible ways to perception, evidence, and all other sources of information reaching the agent. Once the governing ideal of rationality is acknowledged, there also flow from it further restrictions on the ascriptions of the E-concepts at a given time, including holism of explanation by the E-truths at a given time. For example, we have already noted in an earlier section that consistency as a governing ideal of belief is in no way implied by consideration of the *a priori* principle by itself:[27] whereas we are now in a position to rule out attribution of inconsistent beliefs where we do not have any explanation of the agent's failure to see their inconsistency, or do not have reason for believing that there is such an explanation. This also applies to obvious implications of beliefs. And all this further constrains ascription of belief and desire at a given time.

The intertemporal constraint of rationality is clearly not meant to exclude akratic action, and the akrates is irrational. So what do I mean by 'rationality'? First we should note that the intertemporal constraints apply to combinations of beliefs and desires over time, and not to actions. In pure akrasia, there is irrationality in action only. But this observation still leaves a question. For can there not be irrational desires? There are various reasons for calling a desire irrational: that it is not rationally possessed given the agent's underived desires and beliefs, that the agent is not seeing the consequences of fulfilment of the desire even though he has the information to work out those consequences, and so forth. But we have already covered that kind of point: these are all cases that are possible provided there is an explanation of the agent's failure to see the connections.

What of irrational belief? If we can somehow accommodate irrational action and still regard it as intentional, why cannot we accommodate irrationality in belief? We cannot set aside this possibility by the argument that an akratic action at least has its source in some desire of the agent, while there is nothing comparable for irrational belief; for there is indeed something comparable: we can find some small piece of evidence for even the dottiest belief. ('My height is the same as Napoleon's.')

There are some kinds of case in which irrationality in belief does seem unintelligible. Suppose we present someone with something manifestly red in conditions in which he has previously been able to see that red things are red, and he denies that the present object is red. If we want to retain the hypothesis that he is a person to whom the propositional attitude scheme of explanation applies, we must suppose either that there has been some alteration in his perceptual system, or we must alter our account of how he manifests his belief that something is red, or suppose that he does not believe conditions to be normal, and so forth. But this is a specially easy case.

What of the example, given by Michael Bratman in another context,[28] of the woman who irrationally believes that her son has not died in action in Vietnam, in the face of all evidence available to her to the contrary? Is it not silly to insist that in so far as the action explanation scheme applies to her she does not really believe it? What is important here is to see how the possibility of attribution of an irrational belief is dependent upon a basis of dispositions to form rational beliefs. When the mother believes that her son is still alive, her belief would be confirmed for her as well as it could be by her recognizing a certain object as her son, and seeing that he is alive. Implicit in this as confirmation is a large bundle of dispositions to form beliefs of varying strengths that her son is thus and so in circumstances in which someone who seems like her son seems to be thus and so. Moreover, if the woman has a language, the words she uses in expressing her belief are the same ones that occur in sentences that express her rationally formed beliefs. It is hard to see how, if none of this basis of rationality were

[28] In an as yet unpublished paper on akrasia.

present, we would manage to ascribe beliefs to her at all. (Clearly there is a spectrum of cases from the purely rational agent to the insane human being of whom we can make no sense at all.) Anyone interested in further elaboration and development of the claims in this book ought to give as explicit an account as possible of the intertemporal constraints of rationality on the ascription of beliefs and desires: besides their intrinsic interest, the possibility of sophisticated reductions of the E-concepts of the action scheme depends upon their nature.

As a first approximation, we may say that in the perceptual case the intertemporal restrictions are given by the requirement that temporally successive B-truths explained by the scheme must relate to spatially *adjacent* places. The spatial scheme constrains the possible sequences of experiences it explains to those corresponding to *paths* through the space. This is of course consistent with the precise structure of the space – whether or not it is bounded, whether or not it has uniform curvature – being a matter for *a posteriori* investigation.

I have spoken of this as a 'first approximation' because it is not in fact clear that the parallelism requires a restriction to the case in which the motion of the experiencer is continuous.[29] It could be argued that it is *a priori* that there is some restriction, the nature of which is to be empirically discovered, on which places are accessible to the experiencer at a given time interval after he has been at a given place. One argument for this might be that if it were not so, the experiencer could not have empirical reasons for believing that he is at one rather than another of two qualitatively similar places. (His experiences at the next time period together with his theory of the world would not supply such evidence: for if the experiencer's motion is entirely unconstrained, he could have reached a place he knew to be uniquely thus-and-so from either of the two earlier competing places.[30]) I shall not pursue here the issue of how

[29] I should also say that I am not convinced that such a continuity principle is too strong philosophically.

[30] It will be asked: Can there not be indirect evidence via the testimony of others, cannot someone tell the experiencer he was seen at one place and not the other? There are many complications here. One is that the same problem will arise for the testifier if he can move discontinuously too. Another is that it is plausible that the experiencer can establish enough of a theory of an objective world for indirect evidence to be relevant, only if he has already assumed certain

weak the assumptions can be for the parallelism still to hold:
it would certainly be sufficient that it be *a priori* that there is
some empirically discovered restriction that is not in fact
violated too often. For any given scheme of holistic explanation,
we may label as the *holistically connected components* of that scheme
whatever in the scheme is such that the intertemporal constraints of the scheme are given in terms of relations between
those things. Hence the holistically connected components of
the action scheme are the contents of the propositional attitudes
of belief and desires, and those of the spatial scheme are places.[31]
Indeed, it is not incidental to our using just the schemes we do,
that the spatial relations of a given place to other places are
amongst the essential properties of that given place, and that a
particular belief or desire has a certain content.

A perceiver's beliefs about the objective world in which he is
located might be stated, as far as spatial concepts are concerned, solely in terms of spatial relations between particulars
and without use of an ontology of places. How then can I
maintain that the holistically connected components of the
spatial scheme are places? My reply is that a network of spatial
relations between objective particulars, sufficiently rich to allow
the experiencer to distinguish between his own states and states
of the world, seems always to be sufficient to determine some
structure of places at which the particulars are located and
between which spatial relations hold. It is a trivial fact that, if
this reply is correct, the perceiver nervetheless may not have
terms for or variables ranging over places, or in other ways
express beliefs about places. There is no threat to irreducibility
in this, because we have already seen reason in the later part
of section 1 above to hold that even in the crudest kind of
scheme, spatial relations between particulars are, like predications of places, irreducible to appropriate experiential terms.

The intertemporal restrictions on the application of the
E-concepts that we have been considering are to be distinguished
from certain other intertemporal phenomena. For instance, if

restrictions upon his form of motion. (These are complications to be considered
before we begin to think about those arising from the arguments in later sections
that experiences and psychological states must be physically realized.)

[31] This of course does not mean that the relations these constraints require can
be read off from the content specifications alone. Rational patterns of attitudes
will depend on all kinds of background attitudes and dispositions.

we are presented with a persisting object and know that it has some functional goal, then evidence from different times will be relevant to working out simultaneously what that goal is and what the 'ability' conditions of the object are. But once we know what the ability conditions are and what the goal is, there are no further restrictions to be fulfilled. In our cases of holistic explanation, there are further restrictions on the E-concepts even after the ability conditions are known, and these restrictions can rule out some patterns of propositional attitudes, or statements of location and of properties of places, over time. It does not matter whether we compare a term like 'thermostat' with 'person' or with particular E-concepts in the action scheme. If we make the first comparison then the intertemporal restrictions on the application of the E-concepts are additional in the action scheme; if we make the second comparison there are restrictions on acceptable combinations of E-concepts applied to a creature over time that there are not with thermostats. The point that in working out the functional end of an object, we must consider evidence from different times, is really just holism in respect of the evidence again.

How different does all this make holistic explanation from explanation in the physical sciences? The presence of *a priori* principles themselves of course produces a difference from many physical examples. If it really is required that these principles be stated in as explicit a description of mastery of the E-concepts of a scheme as can be given, then it is not possible first to use competently an expression for these E-concepts, and then later to discover that they satisfy these principles; whereas, in contrast, for many physical magnitudes and laws governing them, such a sequence of events is manifestly possible, since it has actually occurred. But this does not by itself produce a difference from all physical examples, and notably not from those in which two physical kinds are simultaneously postulated and linked by a specified principle.

Nor is holistic explanation distinguished by the failure of one-by-one verifiability of applications of the E-concepts that it produces; for this is matched by Duhem's thesis that observations can confirm only sets of hypotheses, and not individual sentences one-by-one. Though Duhem was thinking primarily of generalizations rather than predications of individual objects, it is hard to see why the kinds of arguments he presented could not be applied in the construction of cases in which one-by-one verifiability is impossible without theoretical assumptions about individual objects. (Indeed some of his own examples display that feature.) Nevertheless there is apparently a difference between cases of holistic explanation and examples in which expressions for several scientific magnitudes are simultaneously introduced and in which (as it has to be if there is to be an analogy) it is part of the scientific theory that these magnitudes cannot be identified except by means of their satisfaction of certain principles. The difference is concerned with the point we shall consider in some detail later, namely the existence in schemes of holistic explanation of a familiar distinction between deviant and nondeviant causal chains. (A deviant causal chain in the action case is one in which the intention to ϕ causes the agent to do what he believes to be a ϕ-ing, but in which he does not ϕ intentionally; in the spatial case it is one in which its being objectively ϕ causes the experiencer to have an experience as of its being ϕ, but in which this experience is not a perception.) A full reconciliation of the *a priori* and yet explanatory status of the principles of each scheme will naturally proceed by an account of the realization of beliefs and desires, for instance, in states of matter; and different kinds of explanatory routes from the realizing states to the B-truths explained by the scheme can provide a way of analysing the deviant/nondeviant distinction. In the nature of the physical cases in question it seems there could not be an analogue of this distinction.[32] We will return to this issue in Chapter II (section 5).

[32] In 'Mental Events', after rejecting various other alleged sources as the provenance of the nomological irreducibility of psychological predicates, Davidson writes that 'The point is rather that when we use the concepts of belief, desire and the rest, we must stand prepared, as the evidence accumulates, to adjust our theory in the light of considerations of overall cogency: the constitutive ideal of rationality partly controls each phase in the evolution of what must be an evolving theory' (p. 98). It is hard to believe that a false sentence would result from this if we substituted 'force, mass and the rest' for 'belief, desire and the rest' and 'the unity of physical science' for 'rationality'. I take the suggestions of this section as saying what will (as Davidson surely would) relevantly distinguish the ideal of rationality from those guiding the construction of physical theories. (It is such guiding ideals as the desire for uniformity of operative principles or mechanisms within a given science, that I here intend to cover by 'the unity of science', rather than any reductive construal of this term.)

If this is correct, then we can say generally that three elements must be specified to define a system of holistic explanation:

(1) there is a vocabulary of E-concepts, which appear in
(2) principles that are (a) *a priori* in the special sense noted, (b) causally explanatory in a way we will discuss further below, and (c) contain in their antecedent an unspecified condition C existentially quantified from outside the whole conditional, and
(3) what may be called a *governing ideal* that further constrains the intertemporal application of the E-concepts, the ideal of constrained movement in a system of spatially related places or of the rationality of a pattern of desires and beliefs. This ideal is non-contingently connected with the application of the E-concepts, and produces the special kind of repercussions we have discussed, restrictions upon the temporally successive B-truths explicable by the scheme.

It should be noted that it has not been required for a system of holistic explanation that there be at least two general concepts that feature in the antecedents of the *a priori* principles, in the way that desire and belief, or location at a place and its being ϕ at a place, are such pairs of general concepts: nor was such a requirement invoked to exclude the 'functional' examples. The reason no such requirement has been made is that the important kind of repercussions can be present even when there is only one such general concept. It has, for example, been suggested by Grice and by Grandy that belief is definable in terms of desire:[33] Grandy's definition is (roughly) that x believes that p iff for any q and r, x desires that:

$$(p \supset (q \equiv r)) \supset (x \text{ desires } q \equiv x \text{ desires } r).$$

(These are all desires 'all things considered': intuitively, the suggestion is just that to believe that p is to want your desires to be consistent in the circumstance that it is true that p.) There are many queries that could be raised about the sufficiency of

[33] R. Grandy, 'Reference, Meaning and Belief', *Journal of Philosophy* 70 (1973): 439–52; H. P. Grice, 'Method in Philosophical Psychology (From the Banal to the Bizarre)', *Proceedings and Addresses of the American Philosophical Association* 1974–5, pp. 23–53.

this condition, but let us waive them here, for at present we are interested in the question of what would be the case if some such definition could be given. Let us suppose it could. Then in the *a priori* existentially quantified conditional for the scheme of action explanation, we could replace occurrences of 'believes that *p*' with an expression for the above complex desire, and so the antecedent of the conditional would not then contain a *pair* of general holistically applied concepts. But clearly application of the 'new' complex desires that correspond with conditional beliefs would still be subject to the same intertemporal restrictions; and it would remain the case (as in the arguments against Ayer's kind of reductionism) that no particular action type can be expected to be associated with a desire 'of the form': $(p \supset (q \equiv r)) \supset (x \text{ desires } q \equiv x \text{ desires } r)$, independently of suppositions about the other desires the agent possesses.

Naturally these remarks do not tell against the weaker claim that the antecedents of the *a priori* principles of a scheme must at least state two *applications* of E-concepts, whether this is the same E-concept with a different 'content' in each application (as would be the case if Grice and Grandy are right) or a different E-concept. The weaker claim does indeed seem to be true; and in fact it is unclear how the distinctive feature of the kind of repercussions involved in applying E-concepts could be present unless it were. (It is of course also a requirement that the particular functional example of the thermostat fails to meet. But other cases are not so clear: what of *valve* and *valve-lifter*?)[34]

---

[34] I said at the start that I would not discuss here all the differences and interdependencies between the spatial and action schemes. One such difference consists in the fact that while it seems to be conceivable that beliefs, desires and other attitudes enter into the explanation only of intentional behaviour, it does not seem conceivable that the only explanatory role of 'it's ϕ at p' and 'x is located at p' is in the explanation of experience. I hope it is clear that this difference (significant in other contexts) contradicts nothing I have written here: all I am maintaining is that when applied in the explanation of other kinds of truth, mastery of the spatial concepts has to rest upon the *a priori* principles.

This is an appropriate point at which to note also that I am not excluding the possibility that with great ingenuity in exploitation of higher-order and simultaneous definition someone might come up with a reductive definition of belief and of desire: my position is rather that if this could be done, the definition in order to be adequate would have to identify these states as conforming to the *a priori* principles and the intertemporal constraints on the application of the E-concepts.

It is of interest to consider a scheme that meets all of these requirements other than (2) (b), the requirement that the *a priori* principles in some way be causally explanatory (and consequently it also fails to meet (2) (c)). A good example is provided by the concepts of singular reference and truth-of or satisfaction. This principle:

if a refers to x and F is true of any object y just in case y is ϕ, then the sentence formed from F and a by the predication construction is true iff x is ϕ

seems to have precisely the *a priori* status already discussed. The various suggestions one may make for ways to apply the concepts of reference and satisfaction independently of maintenance of the truth of this principle seem one and all to be defective; and those that are not defective can be shown to have tacitly employed the principle already in a way not explicit in the suggestion but nevertheless essential for the success of the proposed method of application. An instance of the first case would be a man who felt that the truth of a causal theory of reference entitled him to believe there is available a naïve physicalistic reduction of the notion of reference – that is, one ignoring the holism of the psychological and its connections with the semantic – stated in terms of causal commerce between the referent and the state of some part of the human brain. As in the case of the corresponding suggestion about belief or desire, it seems clear that a man with only such a basis for mastery of the concept of reference, with no answerability of the concept to the above principle about reference and predication and all that that involves in its use of the notion of truth, would have no basis for going on to apply the reference relation to creatures with previously unencountered kinds of physiology. Any non-naïve reduction, on the other hand, if it works, will be built in such a way that the above principle comes out true.

What would be an instance of the second case, that in which the basis of application given for the concept is adequate but only because there is tacit use of the principle at some earlier point in the construction? This is provided by those who, inspired by Grice and Schiffer, would provide a definition of reference in terms of the complex of propositional attitudes that must obtain in a community for a reference relation to hold between an expression and an object. Suppose for the sake of argument we accept some such reduction. (The point I am about to make does not exclude the possibility of such a reduction.) Davidson has observed that in radical interpretation there is no attributing finely discriminated propositional attitudes prior to interpretation of the subject's language.[35] It is certain that finely discriminated attitudes would be used in such a definition. Moreover, attribution of these attitudes would surely involve the interpretation of the very expression to which the Gricean definition of reference would be meant to apply. Interpreting that expression is a matter of discovering its reference: and so in applying the Gricean definition we are taken back to a notion of reference subject to the above principle about predication. Of course if a Gricean account is correct, what it is to discover the reference can be explained using nonsemantic terms: but as in the case of non-naïve physical reductions, it will work only if the reductions have the principle about reference, truth, and satisfaction as a consequence.

The condition (3) on schemes of holistic explanation also seems to be met in the reference example. The repercussions of an ascription of reference or a satisfaction condition are consequential upon the way any given singular term(s) can combine with various different predicates, and depend upon the semantic properties of other expressions. Yet it seems clear that even in its very vague formulation the causally explanatory condition (2) (b) I suggested is not met in this example. Obviously one can give a historical explanation of how a sentence in use in a community came to have the truth condition it does, by giving a historical explanation of how its components come to have the semantical role *they* do; but we can do this too for the belief and desire that produce intentional behaviour. The difference rather lies in the fact that the explanation from belief and desire to action seems itself to be causal, whereas it is not causal in the move from reference and satisfaction to truth. The latter is a case of prediction without explanation, comparable in certain limited respects with a rule giving the area of an isosceles triangle in terms of its base

[35] 'Belief and the Basis of Meaning', *Synthèse* 27 (1974): 313.

and height;[36] as the availability of counterfactuals linking height, base, and area shows, such availability is no guarantee of causal connection. The noncausal character of the reference/ satisfaction scheme means there is *a fortiori* no room in it for the presence of 'accidental', 'deviant', or 'irregular' causal connections between the availability of the would-be *E*-concepts and the would-be *B* facts.[37] We will turn to look at this issue of deviant chains in more detail, after redeeming our earlier promise to discuss the relation between our claims so far and doctrines of the absoluteness of space.

5. RELATIONALISM

A question we noted earlier but left undiscussed is this: Is it consistent to accept the irreducibility principles about places and yet not believe in absolute space? That is, is a position that combines a relational theory of space with acceptance of the irreducibility principles a genuine possibility?

In the arguments we have in section 1 above there is a commitment to the view that no particular properties are necessarily possessed by a given place. For if that were not so, it would not be true that the information that someone is located at a particular place is insufficient to settle what kind

[36] Limited, of course, because the concepts of length and height do not have to be applied in accordance with *a priori* principles governing the concept of area.

[37] To forestall misunderstanding, I should add some remarks here about reference and explanation. In *Meaning and the Moral Sciences* (London: Routledge, 1978), Putnam discusses an (alleged) tension between the view that reference is a 'casual-explanatory notion' and the view that attribution of reference, in its role in determining truth conditions of whole sentences, is answerable to the goal of rationalizing behaviour. We are tempted to say it is a causal-explanatory notion because of the attractiveness of the style of realism developed by Richard Boyd, in which it is part of the empirical explanation of the success of the techniques and methodology of a mature science that some of their important theoretical terms refer.

Consider belief: there need not be a physicalist reduction of this, but it is a 'causal-explanatory notion' in the sense that it causally explains *something*, for instance the performance of certain actions. Such *explanandum* sentences will contain physicalistically irreducible vocabulary. Similarly truths containing 'refers to' are causally explanatory of something, viz. the success of certain methods relating to theories (that is sentences used in a language by creatures with propositional attitudes). But this is not to say that reference is *causally* explanatory of the truth of sentences containing the expressions whose reference is in question, i.e., is causally explanatory of a semantic truth, any more than a man's believing something is *causally* explanatory of his holding a certain sentence true.

of perceptual experience he will enjoy there. Let us suppose that it is indeed true that no particular properties are necessarily possessed by a given place. (Certainly, none are *a priori* necessary to it.) It follows that we cannot define location at a given place as the property something has iff it is sameplaced with such-and-such qualitative properties: definitions of this kind will not work in modal and counterfactual contexts. In fact I shall suggest below that not only could any given place at any given time have from that time on wholly different properties from those which it actually possesses: this could even be the case simultaneously for all places at once. If our definitions are meant to work in modal and counterfactual contexts, it is also plausible that we cannot offer definitions of this form either: object x is at place p iff x bears spatial relation R to y and R' to z and R'' to u. Since y, z, and u might be located at places different from their actual locations, something could be located at p without bearing those relations to those objects. (Clearly the condition is not sufficient either.) And to offer a definition in terms of the relation of x to places other than p is to abandon any target of providing a general reduction of the concept of location at a place. All this suggests that if there is to be any eliminative definition of location at a place, it will have to be of a nonqualitative sort and also not make reference to particular objects in the way that the above schema makes reference to y, x, and u.

It will be helpful here to distinguish two notions of absoluteness. (Earman distinguishes at least ten.)[38] The first notion I mention in order to set aside as irrelevant to my present concerns. On this first notion, to claim that space is absolute is to make a theoretical scientific claim. In fact to speak of the absoluteness of space *tout court* is not conducive to clarity: for it has become clear that there can be absolute acceleration without absolute velocity.[39] Let us fix on absolute acceleration. To claim that space is absolute in this respect is to claim that physically there can be motions that can be said to be

[38] 'Who's Afraid of Absolute Space?' *Australasian Journal of Philosophy* 48 (1970): 287–317. The second notion of absoluteness I suggest below is in fact a distinction within his second 'sense'.

[39] For a mathematical exposition of the point, see Earman, op. cit., p. 287; there is a clear intuitive explanation in L. Sklar, *Space, Time and Spacetime* (Berkeley: University of California Press, 1974), p. 205.

accelerations without the need to specify an inertial frame in which they are accelerations. (This formulation is doubly modal because the laws of physics may not require that there be any such motions.) This then is absoluteness$_1$. That space is absolute$_1$ is a claim with the familiar characteristics of theoretical statements of empirical science; it can be experimentally tested in many different ways. Not only are there many different tests in mechanics, but electromagnetic phenomena may also be relevant. Empirical evidence was offered for the absoluteness of space in this sense, and hypotheses which were rivals to those implying the absoluteness of space could have been tested empirically. (The insistence that it is rotation relative to the fixed star shell that produces centrifugal forces could be empirically disconfirmed by an experiment or observation stemming from the possibility of there being an object on which centrifugal forces are acting and yet which is not rotating relative to the fixed star shell.) I shall not discuss these fascinating issues further here: the point at present is that the considerations that make it plausible that location at a place is qualitatively irreducible leave open the pattern of results to be obtained from the sophisticated experiments that would help to settle the question of whether space is absolute$_1$.

The more interesting question is whether the irreducibility principles we have accepted entail the absoluteness$_2$ of space. Absoluteness$_2$ is not implied by absoluteness$_1$. Space is absolute$_2$ iff this principle holds:

(A) The location of events, objects and features at a given time t – which places they occur or are located at – is not fixed (may vary) even though all spatial relations of objects, events, and features to each other are fixed in the following three respects: (i) their relations at t, (ii) their relations at times prior to t, (iii) counterfactuals stated using a vocabulary for spatial relations, but not an ontology of places.

Thus (A) permits the hypothesis of the entire material universe moving with uniform velocity in Euclidean space in a Newtonian universe as a significantly distinct hypothesis from the view that it is stationary: there is a fact of the matter about location in space that all spatial relations fail to settle one way

or the other. It is of this case that Leibniz in his fifth letter to
Clarke wrote: 'There would happen no change, which could be
observed by any person whatsoever' (section 29), and again:
'When there is no change that *can* be observed, there is no
change at all' (section 52). This may be taken as a denial of
(A); and I shall use 'relationalism' as a proper name of the
doctrine expressed by the denial of (A).

The reference to times earlier than t in clause (ii) is not idle
in the statement of (A). The relationalist will hold that it *is*
possible for two alternative histories of the world to have given
common time the same objects and features in the same spatial
relations to one another, and for it also to be the case that in
one history at this time all objects are uniformly one foot to
the north of where they are in the other universe at this given
time: the relationalist will hold that this is possible provided an
appropriate story can be given of how in each history the
successive movements of individual objects has produced this
result from a common earlier stage in the two histories.[40]
Clause (iii) is present because we are interested here in discussing theories about location at places that are so non-
empirical that it is not merely a question that truths about
location are not being settled by what is actually the case, but
are settled when we take into account counterfactuals about
spatial relations between objects; for these theories, location is
not determined even when we take into account those counterfactuals. To assert (A) is to deny that a certain kind of
supervenience holds.[41] The relationalist, one who denies (A)
and so asserts that the supervenience does hold, can consistently
hold that space is absolute$_1$: for the evidence for the absolute-

[40] In section 59 of his fifth letter to Clarke, Leibniz is clear that a relationalist
can allow a somewhat analogous possibility in the temporal case.

[41] If we want to deny (A) and think that the presence of clause (iii) is relevant
to this denial, then this question arises: does this supervenience claim already
require acceptance of an ontology of places, via the principle that true counterfactuals must be grounded in what is actually the case? For discussion of issues
relevant to this question, see M. Dummett, 'What is a Theory of Meaning? (II)'
in *Truth and Meaning: Essays in Semantics*, eds. G. Evans and J. McDowell (Oxford:
Clarendon Press, 1976); Sklar, *Space, Time and Spacetime*, 171–3; G. Evans, 'Things
Without the Mind: A Commentary on Chapter II of Strawson's *Individuals*',
forthcoming in a *Festschrift* for P. F. Strawson; and my own 'Causal Modalities
and Realism' in *Reference, Truth and Reality*, ed. M. Platts (London: Routledge,
1979).

ness₁ of space can come from spatial relations between objects in the important experiments.[42]

It is not at all obvious that there is any entailment from the qualitative irreducibility of talk of location at places to (A); but can we do better than saying 'it is not at all obvious', and actually provide a counterexample to an inference of that form? Here is such an example. Consider our ordinary predications of continuant objects: trees, animals, cars, persons. These may be predications of spatial shape, of how one of these objects was in the past or will be in the future, or of its dispositions to action and reaction. I take it that it is extremely plausible that these predications cannot all be reduced to predications of points, where these predications of points are themselves not sensitive to the spatio-temporal boundaries of the objects in question. 'Predications of points' here means in effect: expressions that Quine would call absolute or relative mass terms.[43] 'Sensitive to boundaries' is used in the sense discussed by Evans.[44] To fix ideas more sharply, let us suppose we have a language L that contains mass terms, absolute and relative, that are not sensitive to the boundaries of particular continuant kinds, as well as predications of continuants; and let L' be a fragment of L that is free of an ontology of continuant particulars and of predicates of them. L' may still contain temporal and causal vocabulary, as well as quantification over times and points. L, we have noted, is plausibly not translatable into its fragment L'. (It should be noted here that this talk of 'continuant particulars' on my part is not meant in any way to be prejudicial to the conception of continuant objects as four-dimensional wholes – nor is it meant to endorse it; the irreducibility claim in question is equally plausible for four-dimensional objects, and it would be sufficient for the argument being constructed that we confine our attention to these alone, regardless of whether they are really what we are speaking of in ordinary language.) The question now is this: Is the following principle (I) plausible?

---

[42] That this combination of views about the two notions of absoluteness is consistent is also implicit in Sklar's remark that even if the aether theory had been confirmed, that would not have made empirically respectable all of the distinctions to which Newton was committed: see Sklar, *Space, Time and Spacetime*, pp. 195–8.

[43] *The Roots of Reference*, section 15, 'Individuation of Bodies'.

[44] See 'Identity and Predication', *Journal of Philosophy* 72 (1975): 343–63.

(I) The truth values of sentences of L relating to a given
   time t that are predications of continuants (i.e., sentences
   in L less L') are not fixed (can vary) even though the
   truth values of all sentences of L' relating to t and earlier
   times are fixed.[45]

(I) does not seem to be true. (Strictly speaking, to show that
the move from irreducibility to (A) in the spatial case is a
non sequitur, we need only show that for *some* such conceivable
L and L', the corresponding (I) is not true.) For example, it is
plausible that although the statement that a particular orange
is spherical cannot be translated into a statement using only
the required kind of predications of points, it seems to be the
case that the totality of true predications of points in the volume
in and surrounding the orange would settle the question of
whether the orange is spherical or not, and the totality of
predications of points over both the given and earlier times
would settle *which* orange is in question: no continuant
difference without some feature-placing difference, we might
say. The features, or predicates of points, it should be noted,
need not be restricted to qualitative ones: 'is acidic', 'is watery',
where the application of these is subject to the general constraints on natural kind terms, may be admitted in L'. Even if
there are legitimate doubts about their admissibility within L',
for our purposes it would in any case be sufficient to consider an
L in which the continuants were not instances of natural kinds:
that would be sufficient to show the inference with which we
are concerned to be a *non sequitur*.

There can be a predicate of points 'lies in a somewhat
flattened orange' or 'lies in a dusty orange'. But then will not
'This point lies in a dusty orange' suffice as a translation of the
non-feature-placing 'This is a dusty orange' or 'This orange is
dusty'? There are two answers to this. First we could restrict
our attention to predicates (of whatever degree) of such a kind
that whether one of these predicates is true of a given n-tuple
of points depends only on the properties of those points, and
not of others. This would exclude 'lies in a dusty orange' (and
also 'ξ and ζ lie in the same dog'). This would be a very

[45] I have not included in (I) a fixing of counterfactuals expressed with feature-
placing vocabulary; the fact that such inclusion is not necessary to make the point
only strengthens the case.

restricted feature-placing language, but as we noted it suffices to give some example in which we have supervenience but irreducibility. The second, more important, answer is this. It may be that for any *given* sentence about continuants, we can invent such predicates of points as 'lies in a dusty orange' (explained, of course, in terms of predications of continuants). But for a significant reduction we must have a finite basis of predicates of points such that for *any* sentence of the continuant language (i.e. for any sentence of $L–L'$) we can translate it into a sentence of L', with just that given finite stock of predicates. And what could this stock be when we consider not only

This is a dusty orange

but also

This is a ripe orange

This is a ripe dusty orange found two months ago at a fruit farm

and so on? There is no way of capturing all of this at once in a finitely based, learnable, feature-placing language.

So in this example, predications of continuants are ineliminable although the truth values of predications of continuants are supervenient on feature-placing sentences. Supervenience and irreducibility are consistently combined. Is the same true in the case of location? Certainly the example of predications of continuants is sufficient to show that the possibility of reduction does not *follow* from the supervenience claim. Still, is it nevertheless true that there is such a reduction?

I will tentatively suggest that there is a reduction of the concept of location as it figures in our prescientific notion of space, which is all I shall be concerned with here. The argument for saying that in this particular case we have not only supervenience but also reducibility is that we establish the locations of objects and events from the evidence of their spatial relations: so if one can acquire knowledge of locations from knowledge of spatial relations, one would expect there to be principles linking spatial relations with location, in accordance with which we judge of location. Now there is no sound general argument from 'established on the basis of such and such facts' to 'reducible to such-and-such facts': there are myriad counter-examples. But I suggest that the example of places has certain properties that differentiate it from the obvious counter-examples to any inference from supervenience to reduction, or (what is not the same) to any inference from certain kinds of statement being evidence to reducibility to that kind of statement.

Consider first the claim that psychological predicates are supervenient on physical predicates, in the sense that there cannot be two situations agreeing in all physical respects but differing in some psychological respect: no one would hold that knowing the physical properties puts one in a position to know the psychological properties – for that can depend upon what the situation feels like from the inside. So there the considerations I suggested in the case of places would not apply. Second, they would not apply in the feature-placing example: for there we can perceive continuants and learn by observation what properties they have. We do not have to reach the knowledge by inference from feature-placing statements. Places on the other hand are not perceptible, and indeed on the prescientific conception of space have no causal influence on objects, events, and persons. This last point also differentiates location from a third sort of case, that of theoretical scientific objects and magnitudes: few would now accept the argument that if all our evidence about electrons is given in observational terms, statements about electrons must be reducible to statements cast in observational vocabulary. But our reluctance to accept such arguments is not independent of our belief that electrons causally interact with the world we do observe. (One can make a corresponding remark separating the case of location to those who hold that our beliefs about physical objects are inferred from statements about sense experience but are not reducible to them.) The fourth case is that exemplified by an example in which, given finitely many data points on a graph, we extra-polate to a curve. Location is not like this either: for in this example the evidence and the conclusion are of the same kind. We move from saying that some pairs of values are correlated to the conclusion that other particular pairs are so correlated; but in the case of location, the evidence consists of statements of spatial relations, while the conclusion concerns not spatial relations between objects or events, but the relations of these to places. Finally there is the case of attribution of sensations

to others, where apparently the gap between evidence and
conclusion seems to belie reducibility to the evidence. But in
the case of location, we have no inclination to say (however
wrongly) that I know from my own case where I am or the
location of other objects. (In the case of some emotions, there
is perhaps a gap between evidence and reducibility even though
there is no temptation to say that I know what it is to have the
emotion from my own case; but in these cases I suspect that
the notion of observation in some circumstances is crucial.)
Without doubt I have not mentioned here all the kinds of case
in which one would reject any move from supervenience or
evidence to reduction, but I hope to have said sufficient to
indicate that the example of location has some very special
features. In the reasons I gave for thinking that location must
be reducible to spatial relations there is no commitment to
some wholesale reductionism.

The position then is that we have some reason for thinking
that a reduction of location must be possible, while knowing
from our earlier considerations that this reduction cannot be
qualitative. The task of giving principles that take us from
spatial relations to locations can be subdivided thus. We need
to supply a method that states how, from a specification for each
time of the spatial relations at that time between objects and
events, a specification of such spatial relations over time, and
a specification of how they could have been, we can move to
statements of location for objects and events: this method
settles for places (1) their identity conditions at a given time,
(2) their identity conditions over time, and (3) their identity
conditions between various possible circumstances. I will give
a very sketchy outline of a programme designed to supply such
a method for our prescientific conception of spatial location.
We will employ the subdivisions just listed.

Let us take task (1) first. For any given time, for each object
(or event – henceforth I will omit this) we can introduce the
place exactly occupied by that object; and we can say that
occupied places p and p' are identical iff for any sortal F, any
F's occupying p and occupying p' are identical.[46] For unoccupied
places we need something more complicated if there is to be

---

[46] But the identity of material objects depends on the identity of places: so is
not the suggestion in the text circular? It would hardly be satisfactory here to

more than one unoccupied place. Intuitively we specify an unoccupied place by the spatial relations something occupying it would bear to other objects. So for each statement of the form 'it is possible that there is some object bearing spatial relations R, R', and R'' to x, x', and x''' (where these variables are assigned three noncollinear objects), we introduce a place. Suppose p is introduced by relations $R(p)$ to the set of objects $S(p)$; and p' similarly for $R(p')$ and $S(p')$. Then we say that places p and p' are identical iff necessarily for any sortal F, if the spatial relations of all actual objects are as they actually are, and are as they actually were in the past, any F bearing $R(p)$ to $S(p)$ and any F bearing $R(p')$ to $S(p')$ are identical.[47] It is clear that a construction guided by such an idea would be adequate only for a prescientific conception of space on which the presence of an additional object does not causally affect the distribution of objects in the space. One way such causal interaction would upset the reductive programme is this. We were aiming to work up to modal identity criteria for places ((3) above) using what we had previously obtained in working on (1) and (2). But if in giving identity conditions at a given time, the actual distribution of objects is sometimes assumed and sometimes not, then we will not be able to answer question (1) until we have a modal ('transworld') identity condition, that is until we have solved problem (3). The procedure would be circular. (It might also be that the laws that determine the nature of the causal interaction of objects on each other presuppose the concept of location.)

The main suggestion I have to make in the second task, the provision of identity conditions over time for places, is that

reply that the suggestion just links various concepts and was not meant to be epistemologically helpful to one who did not already know the identity conditions of places. For the reasons we gave for believing there must be a reduction of location to spatial relations were concerned with how someone could come to know the locations of objects. Rather the reply should be that talk of places is unnecessary in speaking generally of the identity conditions of material objects. Instead of saying that material objects x and y are identical iff there is some sortal F under which they both fall and x and y are located at the same places at the same times, we can say this: they are identical iff there is some sortal F under which they both fall and at all times they bear the same spatial relations (if any) to material objects. This *is* perhaps a condition that one could not apply without some grasp of the identity of material objects: but it does not quantify over places.

[47] The issues raised in n. 41, p. 44 above arise again here.

given two sets of places whose identity conditions at a given time are fixed as above, we identify places over time in such a way as to minimize the total motion of objects between two times. This is vague – are there weighting principles to be used in determining the 'total motion'? – and in some cases will not lead to a unique way of identifying places over time. Nevertheless, one can see that any criterion based on the requirement of minimization of motion will have several attractive consequences. First, if there is no relative motion at all between the two times, there will be no change of place of any object. As an immediate corollary, on this prescientific conception one could never truly say that a universe is moving forward in space with uniform velocity, every part at the same speed. Second, the criterion is nonqualitative: identity over time of a given place is not defined in terms of the qualitative perceptible properties of that place. Third, it can account for some of the revisions of judgements we make in the prescientific scheme. A child brought up on a houseboat will revise his judgements about whether the table has really stayed in the same place when he observes the relations of the houseboat to the rest of the universe: it seems to be relevant to his judgement that on any reasonable way of filling in the details of 'total motion', there is less total motion if one says that the houseboat, rather than the rest of the universe, changes its location.

A natural identity condition for places between different possible circumstances is one stated in terms of branching. Suppose we have two possible histories of the universe, which have a common part up to time t:[48] that is, in these two histories up to t the same particular objects stand in the same properties and relations to each other. After t they diverge. In these divergent branches we can identify places by starting from a place in the common part of the two histories and then keeping track of it in each of the two branches by identifying places at successive times by the criterion of minimization of motion. On the other hand, if two histories have no common initial segment, it seems that identities between places in the two histories are not settled by our prescientific concepts. The branching identity condition makes it clear too that any given

---

[48] I do not mean to imply that the talk of possible histories is ineliminable in favour of primitive modal operators.

place from any given time could have had different properties from that time onwards: in this sense the identity condition is nonqualitative. (Indeed it is arguable that it is intelligible that all places have different histories from a given time onwards: because of some quantum coincidence, almost everything could happen a second later than it actually does. The evidence that it does could come from a clock that records seconds regularly, but may do various different things to record the passing of a second.) But there is still a qualitative trace in the criterion. For if in any case in which places in different histories are identical, those histories have a common initial segment, it follows that such identities will hold only when the places at some time in the past had common properties. But our original intuitions against qualitative reducibility did not go so far as to contradict that.

All these remarks are aimed at the elucidation of a conception of space that we know to be incorrect. That does not make it pointless to study the conception. This is not just because it is only with an understanding of what it replaces that we can see the achievement of any given scientific theory. It is also because one needs to know the structure of this prescientific conception of the world if one is to investigate its relation to concepts of objectivity and – as we are investigating – explanation. Note also that it would be wrong to think that this conception leaves no room for the role of theory in determining what statements of location we accept – for nothing excludes the possibility that theory is used in determining which spatial relations hold between objects. Finally I should note that what I have said can only be a partial account, even of this primitive conception. For in the above I have taken a series of times for granted, while really similar arguments can be applied to the occurrence of an event at a time as can be applied to the location of an object at a place. A full account of the primitive conception would state how locations at places and times and identity conditions of each are determined from a network of spatio-temporal relations between objects.

A natural question to raise at this point is: What, if anything, is the analogue in the action case of the denial of (A) and the nonqualitative reduction in the spatial case?

To obtain any analogue at all, we would need something that

is the analogue of the distinction between places and spatial relations between objects, events, and places. Now given our arguments earlier about intertemporal constraints, in which spatial relations between places played a role corresponding to that of the logical relations between the contents of beliefs and desires, one might reasonably take the analogues of places to be, in the action case, the statements believed. But of course to obtain a thesis that is the analogue of nonreductive relationalism we need also some analogue of things, events, and features that are *at* the places: for it is the relations between these things that are at the places that, according to the denial of (A), in one sense determine the locations of events, features, and objects.

It might be suggested that the intentional actions being produced nondeviantly by beliefs and desires could be the analogues of events, objects, and features being located at places. This would suggest as the action analogue of (A) the following formulation:

(B) What is believed and desired by an agent at time t is not fixed (may vary) even though everything the agent intentionally does, (i) at t and (ii) before t and (iii) would do in various counterfactual circumstances, is fixed.

It is plausible that (B) is false, *modulo* considerations of indeterminacy of interpretation.[49] But it is also not the correct analogue of (A). What an agent intentionally does is what is explained by the *a priori* principles of the action scheme, and what is correspondingly explained in the spatial scheme is the character of a perceiver's experiences. Rather, to obtain a proper analogue we would have in the first place to find something that stands to an agent's belief that if he ϕ's then p as spatial relations between events, states, and objects stand to its being objectively ϕ at p. Perhaps such concepts could be introduced, but the fact that they are not ones we employ in nonphilosophical discourse means that the proper analogue of nonreductive relationalism in the spatial case will not have a pretheoretically intuitive content, and I will not pursue the matter. This is a case in

---

[49] Such indeterminacy would not damage the point, because we could obtain a content common to the various interpretation schemes between which there is no objectively right choice in the way suggested by Hartry Field in 'Quine and the Correspondence Theory', *Philosophical Review* 83 (1974): 200–28.

which we ordinarily employ more of the available structure in the spatial than in the action case and to note this is in no way to cast doubt on the parallelisms already suggested.

I will close this chapter with a disclaimer. Nothing I have written implies that there is some role one can nontrivially specify such that any system of states fulfilling that role is a system of beliefs and desires. What I have said leaves that question open. Certainly if there is such a role it will have to accommodate the feelings and emotions in which desires express themselves. There are many other questions relevant to the view that there is such a role but I will mention just one. The perceptive reader will have noticed that the *a priori* principle of the action scheme remains true if we replace in the consequent alone '$x \phi$'s' by '$x \psi$'s' and prefix the whole principle with a universal quantifier 'for all ψ': for there will be conditions C – though different ones – verifying the existential quantification when the consequent is '$x \psi$'s' just as when the consequent is '$x \phi$'s'. We could specify restrictions on the conditions C to prevent this; but then we could equally specify different restrictions on the conditions that would make false the version with '$x \phi$'s' in the consequent. Since, however, the essence of the holism lies in the intertemporal restrictions on the application of the *E*-concepts, it does not matter if there are these other variant *a priori* principles: the question is whether there are for them intertemporal constraints and some other concept, which correspond respectively to rationality and to the concept of the intentional in the action case. There do not seem to be any. One possible view is that this is so because we have an irreducible idea of what it is to be a rational agent, which cannot be captured in any specification of the intertemporal restrictions on the application of the *E*-concepts that is neutral with respect to which those *E*-concepts are. If that were so, it would be damaging to any view that beliefs and desires are whatever fulfil such-and-such role.

II

DEVIANT CAUSAL CHAINS

There is a distinction between deviant and nondeviant causal chains in both action and perception. An example of a deviant causal chain in the case of action would be a case where an agent has beliefs and desires that make it reasonable for him to ϕ, and which cause him to ϕ, but where he does not ϕ intentionally. A simple instance is provided by a bank clerk who wants more money and knows that he could without detection write some accounts financially favourably to himself, and who is so distracted by this desire and belief that he absent-mindedly writes his own rather than another's name on a line, which action will result in a large payment of money to himself. In the case of perception a deviant chain is present in examples in which although a man's experience as of its being ϕ is caused by its being ϕ, this experience is not a perception: consider for instance a man who, with his eyes open but under the influence of a hallucinogen, is surrounded by redwood trees that produce a scent that causes him to have a vivid visual image of redwood trees which happens precisely to match his surroundings. Although for the sake of brevity I will write about deviant and nondeviant chains *tout court*, in fact deviance is relative to a description. One and the same particular token experience can be an experience as of its being sunny and as of one's being located in front of the White House, and the experience might be perceptual under one of these descriptions but not under the other. (Examples will be given later.)

These two definitions of deviance are not *ad hoc*. They have a common form. Generally, schemes of holistic explanation are definitive of the application of particular concepts in the way that the action scheme is definitive of the notion of the intentional and the spatial scheme of the perceptual. If a scheme S of holistic explanation is definitive of the application of a concept H, then an example of a deviant causal chain in that scheme will be one in which some event (roughly) is (a) caused by certain E-truths appropriate according to the *a priori* principles of that scheme, and (b) is of the kind specified in the consequent of the appropriate *a priori* principle of the scheme *S*, but (c) does not fall under the concept *H*. The definitions we gave in the last paragraph for action and perception are both of this general form.

If the parallel between action and perception that I have claimed really does exist, then we might expect that the basis of the distinction between deviant and nondeviant chains is correspondingly parallel for the two schemes. That is what I shall argue. But the basis I shall suggest for the distinction is one that could be accepted by someone who rejected much of the rest of what I say about holistic explanation, and so it may be of more general interest. In particular, the issue should be of interest to anyone concerned to argue for the view that explanation of an agent's actions in terms of his beliefs, desires and intentions is *some* species of causal explanation. Some writers – Kenny is an example[1] – have taken the existence of deviant causal chains to be a decisive objection to causal theories of rational action. Only by giving a plausible theory of the basis of the distinction in the context of a causal account can such an objection be answered. Similar remarks apply to causal theories of perception.

I . SOME INADEQUATE SUGGESTIONS

Plainly what separates the deviant from the nondeviant chains cannot be the falsity in the deviant cases of such counterfactuals as 'If the belief and desire had been absent, the bodily movement would not have been as it actually was, or would not have existed at all': such counterfactuals are in general *true* in the deviant cases. Nor can we always say that the description under which an event is explained in the deviant cases is different from what one would expect from the beliefs and desires. No doubt the bank clerk did not have the intention to inscribe his name there and then, but in other cases the intention is present and there is such a match with it. If Chopin on some occasion had intended and decided to play the piano as if nervous, and his possession of this plan to play less than perfectly itself so upset him that he played nervously, he would have done

---

[1] *Will, Freedom and Power* (Oxford: Blackwell, 1975), p. 121.

exactly what he intended.[2] Perhaps then it may be said that there can never be a *perfect* match with a given intention to ϕ in these deviant cases, because the intention to ϕ is the intention that one should ϕ as a result of one's possession of this very intention via a nondeviant chain. Now such a view wrongly involves ascribing to anyone with intentions use of a distinction between deviant and nondeviant chains of which he may never have dreamed; but even apart from this, it could not help us here. In these examples the reason that the token actions do not match such intentions is simply that they are produced by a deviant chain. The suggestion gives no clue about what it *is* for a chain to be deviant.[3]

A much more hopeful suggestion is that intentional behaviour is in some way characteristically sensitive to certain facts. One must be very careful in how one tries to sharpen this vague thought. Adam Morton has considered the example of a man, Leo, who thinks that the only way to fulfil his desire to injure a certain other man is to point his pistol north-north-east and pull the trigger;[4] as Leo is preparing to do this, his hand trembles with excitement, the trigger is squeezed and the pistol

---

[2] In this example, Chopin's playing is intentional under the description 'playing the piano' but not under the description 'as if nervous'. It is not always true that if an event is intentional under one of the descriptions specified by the agent's intention, it is intentional under all of the descriptions specified by the agent's intention. A man may intend to raise his hand, and intend to trace out a certain curve in doing so. A nervous state itself caused by his intention may cause horizontal movements of his hand that in fact match his intention: in such an example it could be true that the agent intentionally raises his hand, but the horizontal movements of his hand are not intentional under any description.

[3] The dialectical irrelevance of such a suggestion may be compared with the remark that in some form a description theory of singular genuine reference must be true, because if R is the relation that must hold between an utterance token a and object x for a to refer x, the description 'the object to which a bears R' will be a reference fixing description: this vacuous remark tells us nothing about the nature of R.

It should be clear that it is even more immediately circular to say that the examples so far considered provide no objection to a theory according to which for intentionality of an event under a description, the 'desire to perform an action of type x should result in an *action* of type x' (thus I. Thalberg, *Perception, Emotion and Action* (Oxford: Blackwell, 1977), p. 59). If those events are actions that are intentional under some description, then such a theory simply helps itself to the notion to be explained, that of an event's being intentional under some description, in employing the concept of an action.

[4] 'Because He Thought He Had Insulted Him', *Journal of Philosophy* 72 (1975): 5–15.

happens to be pointing in the right direction. Morton says this is not a case of intentional action because the action was in a certain way not responsive to information:

> For if Leo's information (true or false) about the location of his supposed insulter had changed at the last moment, his time and direction of firing would still have been as they were.[5]

What is the 'last moment' here? Does Morton mean (a) the last moment before (or better: a moment arbitrarily close to) the moment at which the agent decides to fire, or does he mean (b) the last moment before (a moment arbitrarily close to) the moment at which the agent squeezes the trigger? With this question in mind, consider the following example. In any case whatever of human action, an efferent nerve impulse is sent from the central nervous system to the relevant limb. There will be some small finite time interval between the transmission and the start of movement of the agent's body, within which of course the agent can do nothing intentionally to prevent the initiation of the movement. Now consider an example in which this transmitted message is either blocked, drowned out, or destroyed half-way along its path by some neural state that is a result of the agent's nervousness that itself results from the agent's possession of the belief and desire; and we can suppose too that this blocking neural state itself produces by transmission at some later stage of the route a movement of the very type originally intended. (It does not matter whether this is neurophysiologically possible for humans: it is sufficient that it is conceivable in some being to whose actions we would apply the belief/desire scheme of explanation.) Now let us return to the ambiguity in Morton's condition. If Morton meant (a), the last moment before the decision, then the condition he suggests is not sufficient for intentional action, because in our case, though the movement is not intentional under any description, new information received just before the decision may still affect which type of bodily movement is such that a token of that type is produced. If, however, Morton meant (b), the last moment before the movement itself is executed, then the condition is

[5] Ibid., p. 14.

not necessary for intentional action, for in clearly nondeviant cases of action new information at *that* stage is too late to affect which type of movement is performed.

Nor will it help to appeal to the idea of the belief and desire 'controlling' the remainder of the subsequent movement. No such continuation need be intended, as for instance in the case of the man mistakenly taken for dead after some disaster who may intend just to make his hand discernibly move as a sign of life; and anyway the explanation of what it is to 'control' something seems simply to raise our original questions.

All these examples have direct analogues for the case of the perception of things in space that, for fear of tedium, I shall not trace out.

It is extremely natural, and it seems to me ultimately correct, to say that the nondeviant causal chains are those in which the truth of the sentence that forms the consequent of the *a priori* principle for the scheme of holistic explanation in question – that someone ϕ's or has an experience as of its being ϕ – is explained in a favoured, sensitive way by (in the respective schemes) the agent's attitudes or the world being a certain way. The remainder of this section I will devote to an attempt to make more explicit and to sharpen the formulation of this idea of sensitivity. First I shall reject several inadequate explanations of the idea; then I shall give a different criterion for the case of action, and go on to apply it to the perception of things in space.

A first suggestion for explaining that notion of sensitivity might be to say that the mechanism exhibited in a causal chain from certain attitudes to a corresponding movement, does not exhibit the required sensitivity if any stage of the chain it produces could have been produced by entirely different attitudes. The 'could have' here is, superficially at least, non-epistemic. The motivation of this particular initial suggestion is clear enough: the thought behind it is that, for instance, nervousness may be produced by many different beliefs and desires. Thus even though a belief and a desire, or even an intention, may cause nervousness that in turn causes an instance of the intended action-type, the chain is counted as deviant because one of its stages, that of nervousness, could have been produced by many other beliefs and desires (or even by states other than propositional attitudes).

But this suggestion does not work. Consider the later stages of a perfectly normal nondeviant chain. It seems plain that such later stages could have been produced by a sophisticated neurophysiologist with technical apparatus intervening in a man's nervous system at some earlier point (be it centrally or peripherally). The neurophysiologist might even, perversely, produce the later stages of a chain that lead to a movement the neurophysiologist knew his subject had reason not to perform. Of course such a movement would not ordinarily be intentional; the present point is just that the fact that such a case is possible shows that for a chain to be nondeviant it is not necessary that its stages subsequent to the first could not have been produced in any other way, nor by other states of the agent. The requirement is much too strong.

The defender of this first suggestion might appeal to a certain kind of essentialism to meet that objection. He might say there is one – not the only, but one – notion of a state such that if certain facts or events cause an object to be in a certain state S, nothing other than those events and facts could cause that object to be in just that state S. The defender may go on to say that if he uses *this* notion of a state in the formulation of his 'could have' criterion, the objection just raised will no longer go through. This is true. We do not, however, need to stop to assess the plausibility of the implied essentialism about these states in order to see that such essentialism will not help the defender. For if the essentialism about states implies that the stages of a nondeviant chain could not have had other causes, it equally implies that the state of nervousness and its successors in a *deviant* chain equally could not, on that notion of state, have had different causes. The weakening that the appeal to essentialism produces is too great: the criterion it yields fails to characterize obviously deviant chains as deviant.

There are other replies that may be given on behalf of the first suggestion: as, for instance, a requirement that in assessing other possible causes of the stages of a chain we exclude routes that go via the will of another person. I will consider such views later. There are other criticisms that might be made too: how would this first suggestion accommodate the case of a man who becomes nervous in only one kind of circumstance, a Siegfried? For then the 'could have' test wrongly yields, on one reading, the verdict that movements produced by such nervousness are intentional.

Let us turn now to a second suggestion. This second suggestion is that what makes a chain deviant is a certain *independence* of some of its stages from certain truths. Consider the case of the bodily movement which is produced by nervousness caused by the intention to ϕ, and which produces a movement that is a ϕ-ing (or a movement of a kind that would be ϕ-ing if the chain were nondeviant). In this case we may say that the nervousness leads to a bodily movement that is a ϕ-ing quite independently of the fact that a movement of this kind in those circumstances is believed to be a ϕ-ing. In other words, the fact that certain bodily movements are believed to be ϕ-ings has no causal influence on the earlier stages of the chain, particularly the stage of nervousness. Again this suggestion may reasonably claim to express one sense of 'sensitivity'.

The suggestion as it stands is too crude: for it does not pronounce the following case to be deviant, which it is. A man, in contemplating an action, may come to realize that only bodily movements of one particular kind will be instances of his intended action. Because of past associations in his history, the belief that he has to make this kind of movement may make him nervous: and a deviant causal chain from the belief and desire through the intention and the nervousness to an action of the intended kind may be the result. But in this kind of example it is not true that the intermediate stages of the chain are uninfluenced by which bodily movements are believed to be ϕ-ings:[6] for such truths or beliefs do have an influence – they produce the nervousness.

A third suggestion is that the second suggestion was right in appealing to a concept of independence, but failed to elucidate

[6] Where it matters, I distinguish between the agent's intention to ϕ and what he believes to be a ϕ-ing in the circumstances, not because I am not concerned with the final stage of the agent's practical reasoning (on the contrary): I distinguish the two because even at that final stage, there is still a distinction to be drawn. In the example given in an earlier section (p. 13) of an agent whose visual field is (unbeknownst to him) distorted, we can make sense of the idea that the bodily movement he believes will be a stretching out of his arm culminating in reaching the glass will not in fact be a reaching for the glass, even though he (the agent) may not have the concepts to describe without circularity the bodily movement which he does believe will be a reaching for the glass in the circumstances.

that concept correctly. It is this suggestion that I shall develop and tentatively endorse. Of the nervous state in a deviant chain, we may say the following: it has no intrinsic feature F which is both produced by the intention to ϕ, and causally *explains* in the circumstances the production of a bodily movement of just the kind in question, namely, one that is believed to be a ϕ-ing.

There is much here that calls for qualification and elucidation; and, above all, we will want to see a rationale for the need for such an intermediate feature if a chain is to be non-deviant. The initial, crude thought behind the suggestion is that even if the nervousness is produced in the way described in the example given in response to the second suggestion, it is still not true in that example that there is some specific feature F of that nervous state, resulting from the intention to ϕ, which is what determines that the resulting bodily movement is one of a type believed to be a ϕ-ing – as opposed to its determination by other features of the nervous state and by the circumstances that surround the later stages in which the nervousness is transformed into other (in the human case, neural) states. It seems intuitively attractive to say the chain involving nervousness is deviant because the nervous state produces the bodily movement it does only because the circumstances surrounding the later stages of the chain are as they are. But it is obvious that this cannot be by itself entirely the correct reason: for it is equally true in quite central cases of intentional action that good earlier stages of standard chains produce the bodily movement they do only because the circumstances surrounding the later stages of the *nondeviant* chain are as *they* are. More needs to be said. We have in effect a dilemma to avoid. Even if we restrict the application of 'circumstances' to exclude those which can be specified by truths other than those stating that a certain bodily movement (specified physically) is believed there and then to be a ϕ-ing, we can still state the dilemma: if we fail to make reference to the role of later circumstances in the production of the bodily movement, we wrongly exclude some (indeed quite plausibly all) standard chains; while if we bring them in, we wrongly include some deviant ones. We need a somewhat more satisfactory formulation of the intuitive dividing line here.

We may truly say of the nervousness examples that when the state of nervousness does not have features specifically reflecting the intention to ϕ, the circumstances surrounding the chain, by virtue of which the nervousness results in a movement of a kind believed to be a ϕ-ing, hold independently of (are not produced by) the intention to ϕ. Although the bodily movement that results may well be causally determined, it can remain true that it is in a sense accidental that a movement results that is believed to be a ϕ-ing, an accident in the sense that the later stages of the chain from certain attitudes to the bodily movement are determined in their causally relevant features independently of the possession by the agent of these attitudes. A parallel with a certain conceivable kind of camera may help here. Consider a camera containing black and white film. In the causal chain leading to the production of a picture, between the stage of the pattern of light falling on the film and the reaction on the film there is a loss of sensitivity to the colour of the original scene: the state of the film after exposure does not specifically reflect those colours. Now suppose the camera to include a device that reintroduces colour solely from the shades of grey fixed by the state of the film, a device that produces only one colour for any given shade of grey even though many distinct colours may have produced that shade of grey. In some cases the device may produce colours that match those of the original scene. It is then accidental that the final picture matches the scene in the same sense that it is accidental that a bodily movement that is believed to be a ϕ-ing results from the intention to ϕ in the nervousness examples. It may be causally determined that the scene is coloured as it actually is, but even though a statement of matching follows from these two causally determined truths, that is not sufficient for the matching to be nonaccidental in our present sense: for that, one must cause the other (or they must have a common cause) via the right kind of causal route. We still have not said what that route is.

2. DIFFERENTIAL EXPLANATION

I plan now to proceed as follows. In the cases of deviant causal chains we have a failure of what I shall label 'differential explanation' to hold between certain truths and certain other truths. I will give two examples of failure of differential explanation in areas distinct from action and perception, and then go on to give a brief account of what is involved in differential explanation.

First, consider that camera with the colour reinsertion device. Let us take it as it is, and add yet another device to it. We add a second light- and colour-sensitive device, which operates a second shutter; this shutter opens only if a certain definite total pattern of colours in the surrounding scene is picked up by this light- and colour-sensitive device: the pattern might be that determined by a foursquare view of the Doge's Palace at noon in May. Let us call this camera 'the second camera': this is now a camera that has two shutters, one of which is linked to the new device, and it too contains the colour reinsertion mechanism. Then it is true that the particular pattern of colours in the scene, and nothing weaker, enters the explanation of the distribution of colours in the picture produced: in this respect it of course differs from the first camera, in which citing the distribution of colours involves some redundancy – the explanation there need cite only the distribution of light classified according to the shade of grey it produces. Nevertheless, in the way I am using the term, the distribution of colours does not differentially explain the pattern of colours in the picture produced by the second camera (unless we suppose, as we do not, some mechanism linking the scene and the grey-to-colour conversion device). If there were a putative perceptual mechanism working on lines similar to that of this second camera, then an experience produced by it would be perceptual under descriptions specifying the shapes and arrangement of objects in the original scene, but not under descriptions specifying their colours.

Some may be tempted to remark of this example that they do not agree that the distribution of colours in the scene explains the distribution of colours in the photograph taken by the second camera: the distribution of colours in the external scene explains the opening of the second shutter, and thus in the circumstances explains why some picture was taken, but in the case of a camera like this, the external distribution of colours does not explain the details of the particular picture produced. It is not to be denied that we sometimes use 'explains' in this way. But it is also clear that when we do so, 'explains' means more than 'is a nonredundant part of the total explanation of': what more is involved is the object of our search, and the correct remark about the use of 'explains' does not by itself bring us nearer that goal.

Other examples of the failure of differential explanation to hold as a relation between certain truths can be constructed by taking the second camera's additional shutter as a model. In normal surroundings, the pattern of nucleotides in the DNA molecules that constitute genes differentially explains a vast range of the characteristics of the human being that develops in accordance with the instructions they encode. But it is not inconceivable that in the future a biochemist should be able to place a gate, as it were, across the route of development from the genes to the final product so that only genes that were tokens of a fully determinate type would find their instructions implemented, for only tokens of this type would pass through the gate. If such a gate were in operation, but, owing to unfortunate (or fortunate) later conditions, not all aspects of the encoded plan were chemically implemented, then the following could be true: in the explanation of why the organism is as it is, the fact that its genes are tokens of the given type plays a nonredundant part – for if it had not had genes of this type, there would have been no organism at all. Nevertheless the complete specification of this type does not differentially explain in such circumstances the characteristics of the organism. (Note that the organism by a fluke might in fact be of exactly the same kind as it would have been if all the components of its genetic programme had been implemented under standard conditions, the conditions genes of that kind had evolved to cope with.)

It is evident that what is involved in differential explanation needs for its statement finer distinctions than a simple use of necessary and sufficient conditions can supply. For in cases where we do have differential explanation, what differentially explains is not by itself sufficient for what is so explained (the distribution of colours in the external scene differentially explains the colours of the picture in an ordinary camera, but the film needs to be working); while equally a condition that fails to differentially explain may be necessary in the circumstances for what is explained.

The simplest case in which we can draw the finer distinction that is relevant for us is one in which we have a law (or a derived law, or, more generally, any acceptable explanatory principle) of this form, where 't' ranges over times and 'n' over numbers and '$k(\ )$' is some numerical functor:

$$\forall x \, \forall t \, \forall n (Fxt \,\&\, Gxnt. \supset Hxk(n)(t + \delta t)).$$

Suppose we have as *explanans* that Fxt and $Gxnt$ for some particular x, t, and n. These conditions are jointly sufficient and severally necessary for the *explanandum* $Hxk(n)(t + \delta t)$: in these respects the two conditions are symmetrically related to the *explanandum*. Nevertheless we may say that the differential explanation of x's being H to degree $k(n)$ at the time $t + \delta t$ is that it was at t G to degree n, just because according to the principle of the explanation invoked there is a functional connection between the two, expressed by k.

More generally, we may offer this rough definition: x's being ϕ differentially explains y's being ψ iff x's being ϕ is a nonredundant part of the explanation of y's being ψ, and according to the principles of explanation (laws) invoked in this explanation, there are functions (such as k in the above example) specified in these laws such that y's being ψ is fixed by these functions from x's being ϕ. There are at least two possible sources of misunderstanding to be noted here. The first is that the gerund 'x's being ϕ' is not to be taken as referring to some entity in the world (relative to an assignment to 'x'). 'Differentially explains' is of the same category as 'explains' itself: it is an operator that takes a pair of sentences (closed or open) to yield a sentence that is open if at least one of the sentences on which it operates is open. 'x's being ϕ' is just a convenient form in which to indicate the sentence on which 'differentially explains' is operating. Any adequate extension of Davidson's paratactic account of the logical form of sentences of indirect discourse to include relational indirect discourse will be applicable to 'differentially explains' too.[7] A second possible

---

[7] D. Davidson, 'On Saying That', *Synthèse* 19 (1968): 130–46; for one extension of Davidson's theory to the relational case see J. Hornsby, 'Saying Of', *Analysis* 37 (1977): 77–85.

misunderstanding should be ruled out if we note explicitly that 'fixed' adverts only to the uniqueness of determination by the function (as a matter of mathematics in numerical cases): it does not imply that the laws are not statistical.

The functions specified in the laws invoked in an explanation may be defined not only over numbers but also over colours, chemical elements, compounds, shapes, and so forth. It should be clear how this is relevant to our more recent examples. In the case of the picture produced by the second camera, a sentence stating the distribution of colours in the external scene is a nonredundant part of the *explanandum* consisting of a sentence which stated, using presumably elementary mathematical apparatus, the distribution of colours in the picture produced: but it is not the case that any operative principle of explanation makes that second distribution of colours a function of the first – it is determined rather by the function obtained by the operation of the colour conversion device applied to the distribution of light classified by the shades of grey it produces on the film before the colour conversion device operates. Analogous remarks apply in the genetic example.[8]

In all the examples given so far, the condition that differentially explains has been one of a set of conditions such that, given the same principle of explanation employed in the particular case in question, then if similar conditions had been met by other objects at other times, a corresponding *explanandum* sentence would be true: the set of antecedent conditions is strongly sufficient. There are important kinds of empirical explanation where such strong sufficiency is absent, but the kind of functional connection involved in other cases of differential explanation remains present, and we will still apply the latter concept in such cases. John Mackie considers the example of a chocolate machine he labels '*L*' which will 'not in normal circumstances produce a bar of chocolate unless a shilling is inserted, but it may fail to produce a bar even when

---

[8] In the treatment of these examples, we are of course relying heavily on an 'explains' relation that takes a pair of sentences to form a sentence, rather than on a causation relation between token events (things in the world). To this extent, I regard the terminology of 'deviant causal *chains*' as unfortunate: for it is not properties of the events themselves but rather more complex conditions relating to the *principles* of explanation that I am claiming to be the basis of the distinction.

this is done'.[9] We might consider a similar machine, which produces a different size of bar according to the value of coin
inserted: we may be in a position to say that its production of
a bar of a specified size is differentially explained by the value
of the coin inserted, there being a listable functional relation
between coin value and size of bar produced, without any
implication that the differentially explaining condition is an
element of a set of conditions strongly sufficient for the production by that machine of a bar of that size. (Admission of this
case will be important in the application of this distinction.)

There are two restrictions I shall take to be in force when
one condition differentially explains another. The first is that
the covering law of the explanation must be a causal law:
instances of the antecedent must cause instances of the consequent. The second restriction is perhaps implicit in the notion
of a law, and it is that the law be written in a form without
redundancy and using projectible predicates (or mutually
projectible predicates). Otherwise we can make anything a
function of anything by logically equivalent rewritings. Both
these two restrictions are evidently highly problematic, but they
are general problems rather than problems for my account
alone; and many different solutions to them would be consistent
with the theory of deviance I will be offering.

'Differentially explains' is a transitive relation: that follows
simply from the fact that if x's being F differentially explains y's
being G and y's being G differentially explains z's being H, then
in effect by taking the composition of the two functions that
verify these two relations, we obtain a function that verifies that
x's being F differentially explains z's being H. More important
for us is the fact that under simplifying assumptions, the converse is also true. Suppose (as is not true generally, but may
hold locally of particular systems of objects) that we can divide
time into intervals, such that at each interval, any state of the
world that is causally produced at all is causally produced by
the state of the world at the previous time interval. Now
suppose that x's being F at interval t differentially explains z's
being H at interval $t + 2$. Under these assumptions, we must
have that for some object y and for some property G, x's being

[9] J. L. Mackie, *The Cement of the Universe* (Oxford: Clarendon Press, 1974), p. 41.

F at t differentially explains y's being G at $t+1$, and that in turn differentially explains z's being H at $t+2$. For if that were not so, then under these assumptions, whatever z's being H at $t+2$ is a function of according to the operative principles of explanation, it will not be a function, by those principles, of x's being F at interval t. This has the following implication for any system that fulfils the assumption about intervals: if the state of one object at one time is to differentially explain the state of another object at a later time, then at every intervening time interval there must be some object in some state G such that its being in state G is differentially explained by, or as we may conveniently say for the converse of this relation, *specifically reflects*, the fact that the first object was in the state it was at the first time, and its being in state G also differentially explains the final object in question being in the specified state. There must be a chain of such features or states of the intermediate stages for a claim of differential explanation to be true. This is not to say that to *know* such claims to be true we have to know what these intermediate features are: at most we need to know that there *are* such features. When there are such features, we may say that the chain is *sensitive*, relative to an initial object's being in a certain state.

It will no doubt have been evident for some pages that I am going to claim that for a chain from the intention to ϕ to a bodily movement believed to be a ϕ-ing to be nondeviant, the agent's possession of the intention to ϕ must differentially explain his bodily movement of a kind believed by him to be a ϕ-ing (and differentially explain it under that description, of course).[10] The sense of this claim is not immediately clear, since it is not obvious what it might mean to talk of something's being a function of an intention, according to the operative principles of explanation. I shall take for granted in this section a principle the content of and evidence for which I shall consider in a later chapter, viz. the principle that every psychological state in which a given person is at some given time, is realized for that

---

[10] Note that if this is correct for schemes of holistic explanation generally, then we have a 'transcendental' derivation of the principle that a scheme of holistic explanation can be applied to a field of phenomena only if certain parts of it are governed by laws, possibly of a statistical kind: without such laws there can be no differential explanation.

person at that time by some physical state.[11] Now for differential explanation in nondeviant action chains, a bodily movement of a kind believed to be a ϕ-ing is differentially explained (under its bodily movement description) by the neurophysiological state that realizes for the given agent at the given time his psychological state of intending to make a bodily movement of a kind he takes to be a ϕ-ing in the circumstances (for a specific substitution for 'ϕ'). (Many refinements are possible here but this gives the general requirements.) In the case of someone 'acting' out of nervousness, his bodily movement is differentially explained not by the physiological realization of his intention, but by the physiological states with which the nervousness interacts to produce a bodily movement that may just happen to match his original intention, but which is no function of the intention (its neurophysiological realization) according to the principles of explanation involved.[12] Note that since realization is relative to an agent and a time, and since agents vary in their beliefs about how to ϕ, for a given ϕ it will not always be the *same* law that covers the explanation of the bodily movement when the chain is nondeviant. The law can vary from person to person, and will often be a law stated at the electrochemical level.

A rational agent might be such that his internal physiology has the property that there is a probabilistic element in the chain from certain intentions to action; perhaps in 50 per cent of cases the intention is realized, and in 50 per cent chaotic bodily movement results. Here one's intuition is that this fact need not prevent the appropriate bodily movements from being

---

[11] Given the use made of this assumption in the next sentence of the text, it should be clear that a principle about realization and not supervenience is what we need. Even if the state upon which a psychological predicate supervenes is finitely specifiable, it can still be that (a) there is no finite or recursively enumerable specification of all the circumstances upon which the given predicate will supervene; and more to the present point (b) other psychological predicates – perhaps certain beliefs – may also supervene on the given physical description upon which the intention supervenes. In that case to require as we do specific reflection of *that* physical state would be much too strong; while on the other hand, given only supervenience, there may be no more restrictive physical state upon which the intention supervenes but nothing else does.

[12] Note also then that according to the conditions proposed here, we do not have intentional action if the kind of nervousness that results in any given circumstances specifically reflects the agent's intention to ϕ but no feature so reflecting the agent's intention is causally influential on later stages of the chain.

intentional when they do result (in roughly half of the cases). The earlier admission that what differentially explains need not be strongly sufficient for what is differentially explained means that this intuition is not incompatible with the account in terms of differential explanation. In the nonchaotic chains sensitivity as defined above may be preserved.

When we drop simplifying assumptions, the converse of transitivity need no longer hold for differential explanation. We might have an example like this: the intention that the agent has at time t gives rise to two causal chains. One of them produces a state in the agent that starts to hold from $t+1$ onwards, the other producing at $t+5$ a triggering event which may be the same for many different intentions, but which together with the other persisting state caused by this particular intention, leads to a bodily movement of the kind the agent intended. In such a case, even though the triggering is not specific to the particular intention in question, provided the state on which it acts is so, then the condition of differential explanation of the action under the relevant description by the intention is fulfilled.

I do not claim that this account of differential explanation and its application will not need a great deal of refinement and qualification (I am sure it will): here I want only to claim that its materials will function as the core of any better revision. We will later find some confirmation for this in its analogue for the case of the perception of things in space; but before I turn to that I shall make a few more comments on the distinction and its application.

Differential explanation may be preserved by all kinds of unusual re-routings of the causal chains involved in action, and when it is so preserved, intentional action will be produced.[13] This holds not only of such traditional prosthetic devices as artificial limbs but also in more recherché cases. If a man after some brain injury were unable to realize his intentions because of some blockage in his central nervous system, it is not absolutely inconceivable that a surgeon should re-route standard chains in a way that involved a device in one part of the brain transmitting radio signals, and another part receiving and

[13] 'unusual': *pace* A. Goldman, *A Theory of Human Action* (New York: Prentice-Hall, 1970), p. 61.

transforming these signals; the states of these objects could be differentially explained in the right way, and if they did it seems wrong to deny that this man acts intentionally when such mechanisms are operative. It seems clear that in other respects he could be like any other human being. I am not therefore in agreement with those who would require that, for a bodily movement to be intentional under some description, the route from intention to movement should not pass outside the agent's body. It seems obvious too that a variation of the example shows it to be too strong to require that no physical object outside the agent's body may play a role in the causal chain: perhaps an external and separate 'boosting' device increases the radio signal before it is picked up by another part of the brain. Those who maintain the bodily requirement might say that in this case the external device is really part of the agent's body. But if they do say this, it is clear that what they count as part of the agent's body is being determined by the route followed by already identified nondeviant causal chains, rather than conversely.

Is the criterion rather much too strong, and not really necessary for intentional action? One reason that might be offered for that view is this: a man may realize that the only hope he has of performing a certain 'act' is to make himself so nervous that he then, in the circumstances, acts wholly as a result of nervousness. So he takes a drug that makes him nervous, and then acts in the desired way, and achieves his ends in the way planned by him. Do we not have here intentional action without fulfilment of differential explanation? Here one's first intuition, which may not be incorrect, is to say roughly this:

The token event that is his bodily movement is not intentional under any description: this is of course not to say that (*ceteris paribus*) he cannot be held responsible for it, since he may have chosen, as he did in our example, to place himself in that state knowing its likely consequences. Nor is it to deny that the movement was intentional in some weaker, second-level sense, viz. that it was the planned consequence of something that was intentional in the primary sense (swallowing the drug); but that is not enough to make it intentional in the primary sense.

But there is perhaps a better treatment of cases in which account was taken by the agent in his plan of the likelihood of nervousness, a treatment I will mention but leave for further consideration rather than endorse here. Consider the following case. As Freud's servant I form on Monday the intention to break the master's vase on Wednesday when I pick it up. Call this intention i. But I also know that I, and everyone else like me in such circumstances, will become extremely nervous once the vase has actually been picked up. I know too, we are to suppose, that an inevitable consequence of such nervousness is a loosening of the grip and a smashing of the vase. So I know that intervening and operative nervousness will not prevent attainment of my goal. On Monday I decide also, since I am bad at remembering how my more devious plans are meant to work, that I must continue to have an ordinary intention to break my master's vase throughout Tuesday and Wednesday until it is the appropriate moment on Wednesday for it to become operative. (I also lose the knowledge about the intervening nervousness and its effects.) I am successful in continuing to have the intention of breaking the vase in the normal way up to the relevant time on Wednesday, when I pick up the vase and then drop it out of nervousness. Now suppose intentions are 'individuated' not only by their content, but also by when they are possessed (and perhaps by more too); and let us call my intention of Wednesday to break the vase in the normal way 'i'''. (Again, I do not take the apparent quantification over intentions to be ineliminable.) Was the event e of my releasing my grip intentional or not? When we reflect both upon what actually happened, and my quite reliable plan of Monday, we can no more give a non-relative answer to this question than we can to the question 'Is New York north?' when there is no tacit fixing in some way or other of some place relative to which the question is being asked. We ought to say that e is intentional with respect to intention i but not with respect to intention i''.[14] The view that 'is intentional' is a relational predicate (expres-

---

[14] Strictly, we should say that the suggestion is that the two-'place' 'e is intentional under description ϕ' is to be replaced with the three-'place' 'e is intentional under description ϕ with respect to intention i'. One difference between this suggestion and that of the previous paragraph is that under the latter, my dropping of the vase as Freud's servant is not literally intentional under any description at all.

sion) dovetails neatly with the account of the deviant/nondeviant distinction in terms of sensitivity and differential explanation. On that account nondeviancy is, roughly, a matter of the nature of the causal chain from intention to event, and it is clear that a chain from one intention can have the features and a chain from another intention not possess them. There is no deviancy of chain from the original intention i of Monday because from the point of view of that intention the anticipated nervousness plays a role in the agent's practical reasoning analogous to that played by an anticipated crosswind in a helmsman's practical reasoning about the angle at which to hold the tiller. We tend to overlook, the suggestion would go, the fact that 'is intentional' (in the sense in which it abbreviates 'is intentional under some description') is further relative to an intention, just because normally only one intention is in question.[15]

Let us turn now to perception. The criterion I have given for nondeviancy of chain in the action case has a natural and attractive analogue in the perceptual case. It is simply that for an experience as of its being ϕ to be really of its being ϕ, its being ϕ must differentially explain the occurrence of the experience event under the description 'experience as of its

[15] Care in specifying the description under which an event is intentional sometimes simply dissolves some alleged problems. *Analysis*, 'Problem' number 16 (March 1977), set by R. J. Butler, was this:

'If Brown in an ordinary game of dice hopes to throw a six and does so, we do not say that he threw the six intentionally. On the other hand if Brown puts one live cartridge into a six-chambered revolver, spins the chamber as he aims it at Smith and pulls the trigger hoping to kill Smith, we would say if he succeeded, that he killed Smith intentionally. How can this be so, since in both cases the probability of the desired result is the same?'

The alleged problem simply arises from not comparing like with like. The shooter has control over the conditional that if the gun fires, then it fires in one direction rather than another. But he does not have control over whether the gun fires at all. So we say that he intentionally shot Smith, but not that it was intentional of him that a full rather than an empty chamber was engaged. Now in the dice case, the agent has control over whether, for instance, the die falls on one side of the table with the six uppermost *if* it falls with the six uppermost at all, but he does not have control over the antecedent of this conditional. We say in this case exactly what we would expect to say by analogy with the gun example: it may be intentional of the agent that the die falls on the left-hand side of the table, but not that it falls with a six uppermost. Butler's problem arises only when we compare a condition over which the agent does have control in the gun case with a non-corresponding condition in the dice case over which he does not have control.

being ϕ'. The attractions of such a suggestion are straight-forward. The case of the scent-producing redwoods does not yield an experience that is really a perception of its being ϕ because what differentially explains the experience of the specific kind actually produced is some past memory, some half-remembered dream or picture, in any case something other than the redwood trees being arranged in such a corresponding configuration around the experiencer.[16] The requirement of differential explanation also properly excludes an example suggested by Strawson: that of a hallucinating man who hallucinates a brain that matches his own brain which is of course (in a broader sense than that required by my criterion) causally involved in the generation of the hallucination. In such a case there are no features F of the intermediate brain state stages nor of the final experience that specifically reflect, are differentially explained by, the fact that the brain is thus-and-so, grey and damp, say. Strawson himself has a different explanation of the failure of the hallucinating brain to yield perception of the brain that is hallucinating; I will return shortly to discuss his account.

Some may be tempted to offer a different reason for denying the title of perception to the experience in these examples, viz. the falsity of certain counterfactuals. For example, if one of the trees in the clump of redwoods were to move, there would be no corresponding change in the experience; if the hallucinating brain changed colour or shape there need be no causally induced change in the experience; and so forth. I will label as a 'counterfactual theory' any theory to the effect that there is a certain collection of counterfactuals the holding of which is necessary and sufficient for nondeviance. There are three preliminary remarks to be made before I discuss such theories. First, if explanation itself can be defined in terms of counter-factuals, then of course the correctness of the differential explanation theory will imply the correctness of some counter-factual theory. My point will be just that the particular

---

[16] The criterion also covers the case of Kinglake's hallucination cited by Strawson (in 'Causation in Perception' in *Freedom and Resentment and Other Essays* [London: Methuen, 1974], at pp.77–8) in a specially pleasing way if Kinglake's diagnosis (p. 78, footnote) was correct: Kinglake wrote that the heat, dryness, and stillness had rendered his hearing organs 'liable to tingle under the passing touch of some mere memory'.

counterfactuals that have been suggested, which are much more specific than those that might be derived from some general account of explanation, should not feature in a theory of deviance. Second, nothing I will say tells against a counterfactual theory of causation – what I say here is neutral on that issue. It is evident that if a counterfactual theory of deviance is correct, the counterfactuals that discriminate the cases must be other than those true just because a causal claim is correct, since *ex hypothesi* we have causation in both the deviant and the nondeviant examples. Third, I am not denying what is obviously correct, that very often counterfactual sensitivity is found in nondeviant cases and is absent in the deviant ones.

Nevertheless there are cases on which counterfactual theories and the differential explanation account pronounce differently, and where the differential explanation theory marches in step with our intuitions. Let us consider first the non-necessity of counterfactuals for nondeviance. Suppose that a person perceives an array of objects in a television studio which is insulated from all outdoor light. We can suppose too that these objects affect light-sensitive devices which are connected to the studio lighting in such a way that if any one of them perceptibly moved or visually altered, then all the lights would go out and nothing would be perceived. Hence it would not be true that if any one of the perceived objects altered, there would be a corresponding change in the person's experiences. But this does not in any way throw doubt on the claim that the person in the studio perceives the array of objects: it is a clear case of perception. This example can be adapted to raise questions for any counterfactual theory. It would not help, for instance, to say that the counterfactuals that matter are those to the effect: if any of the objects in the array were to alter, then *if* the person experienced anything, it would be a correspondingly altered experience. For that would not be true if, for instance, an alteration in one of the perceived objects caused the release into the air in the studio of some hallucinatory drug. The underlying intuition in these examples is this, crudely expressed: it does not matter what contraptions fill the studio, and how they may affect the truth of various counterfactuals – what matters is how the experience is *actually* related to the array of objects. My own intuitions about the example do not make the presence of the normal mechanism of perception crucial to it. Allowing, as I would, that someone can see with a television camera in place of an eye, or a device bypassing a blocked optic nerve, I would not find it intuitive to say that someone with such a prosthetic visual device sees when he is outside the studio but not when he goes inside it.[17]

There are also questions about the sufficiency of counterfactual sensitivity for nondeviance. To raise the questions we can alter and refine our redwood example. Suppose that the man amongst the redwood trees happens to have a stock of memory images, each one of which is qualitatively similar in content to an experience he would have if he were perceiving one of the patterns that the branches of the redwoods around him might make. Suppose, too, that every such possible pattern has a qualitatively similar memory image. Finally, suppose that each type of image that falls on his retina activates into an experience the contents of a given memory cell; and it so happens – by causes unrelated to the surroundings of our person – that for each type of image which may fall on his retina, the memory image in the cell whose contents it triggers is qualitatively similar to the triggering image. In such an example there may be as great a degree of counterfactual sensitivity to the external scene as there is in normal perception. My own intuition is that this is still not a case of perception, and those with this intuition can again conclude that the line

[17] The studio example also shows the differential explanation account to be different from H. H. Price's well-known distinction between 'standing' and 'differential' conditions (see *Perception*, 2nd edn. (London: Methuen, 1950), p. 70). In the course of his formulation of the causal theory, which he unfortunately never separates from the false claim that perceptual knowledge of external objects is essentially inferential, Price says that standing conditions are those 'necessary to all the visual sense-data alike'. This condition is underspecified: is what is in question all the visual data of a given occasion, or all the visual data ever of a given perceiver? Grice reads Price the former way and objects that Price's use of the distinction is not sufficient to cover all cases ('The Causal Theory of Perception', *Proceedings of the Aristotelian Society*, suppl. vol., 1962); and it is also not necessary because the whole of my visual field may be taken up by a uniformly coloured wall without it being false that I see *it*. On the particular-occasion construal of Price, the inside studio scene being as it is may be a *standing* condition in Price's sense, and so he would wrongly fail to count this as a case of perception.

The non-particular-occasion construal of Price yields an even more implausible theory; since the operation of the generator in another room is not a causal precondition of *all* my visual sense-data, the standing/differential condition would not exclude that the generator was perceived.

between perception and nonperceptual experience depends not upon counterfactuals, but upon how the experience is actually related to what explains its occurrence. A different reaction to this example might be to say that what we have in it is a temporary and fortuitously acquired perceptual mechanism. (David Lewis suggested to me such a response.) I will discuss such a reaction later. Perhaps for now it is worth noting that counterexamples to the necessity of counterfactual sensitivity for nondeviance can be seen as more important than counterexamples to sufficiency, since if we do not have necessity then counterfactuals will not be part of a uniform account of nondeviance.

It may be asked: how *can* the differential explanation and the counterfactual theories come apart? Does not the differential explanation theory speak of functions referred to in covering laws, and must not these laws sustain counterfactuals? Here we need to distinguish two classes of counterfactuals. There are the counterfactuals of the kind we have been talking about in discussing counterfactual theories, and there are those sustained by the covering laws just mentioned. We can illustrate this distinction even in our extremely simple case in which the covering law was

$$\forall x \, \forall t \, \forall n (Fxt \,\&\, Gxnt. \supset Hxk(n)(t + \delta t)).$$

If a particular object x is H to degree $k(n)$ at $t + \delta t$ because it was F and was G to degree n at time t, then, we noted, one could say that x's being H to that degree at the later time was differentially explained by x's being G to degree n at the earlier time. The two different counterfactuals we should consider (where we use '$\square\!\!\rightarrow$' for the counterfactual conditional and where m is some number distinct from n) are:

(i) $Gxmt \;\square\!\!\rightarrow\; Hxk(m)(t + \delta t)$

and

(ii) $Gxmt \,\&\, Fxt. \;\square\!\!\rightarrow\; Hxk(m)(t + \delta t).$

In the circumstances as we have described them, there is no guarantee that the counterfactual (i), which is the analogue here of the counterfactuals offered by counterfactual theories, is true: for it might be that if x had been G to degree m, then it would not have been F. Counterfactual (ii) on the other hand will be true in these circumstances. Does this mean, then, that counterfactual theories will be safe from these objections provided that they appeal to counterfactuals on the model of (ii)? But the problem then for the counterfactual theorist is how he is to unify the antecedents of the counterfactuals which he does count as relevant to nondeviance from one occasion to another. Which are they? The theorist of differential explanation is going to say that they can only be unified as counterfactuals the antecedents of which are drawn from laws covering a differential explanation, and if this is correct, it prevents any collapse of differential explanation into a counterfactual theory.

Does what we have already said about differential explanation capture the intuitions about sensitivity with which we set out? There are some reasons for thinking that it does not. First, the function that is mentioned in the covering law in an example of differential explanation may be very far indeed from one-to-one: it seeems reasonable to want more than this if we are meant to be capturing a notion of sensitivity that does not involve loss of a certain structure in transmission. Second, if indeed an ordinary camera displays the kind of sensitivity in which we are interested and the second camera we described does not, then the account so far of differential explanation is not complete: for in the case of the second camera, there *is* a function by which the distribution of colours in the final picture produced is determined by the distribution of the colours in the original scene. This will be the function determined in part by the principles of operation of the colour-conversion device. It would not do to reply to this that what matters in differential explanation is that what is differentially explained is a function only of arguments mentioned in what does the differential explaining. That would not be true in the case of a normal camera: the picture produced there is also a function of the distribution of the densities of the glass in various parts of the lens, and so forth. These considerations suggest that more restrictions are needed.

I suggest that what we have to add to the weak differential explanation already defined is a condition of recoverability. I will say that p *strongly* differentially explains q if p differentially explains ('DE's') q in the sense already explained, and given the initial conditions of the explanation (of q) other than p, together with the fact that q is the explanandum, one can recover (work out) the condition p. Such recoverability is certainly present with an ordinary camera: given details of the film, lens, camera size, and so on, and the laws of motion of light and its effects on the film, one can work out what distribution of light must have produced just the picture that resulted. This recoverability restriction accommodates two points we were missing with weak DE: under strong DE, the function, in some circumstances we discuss below, will need to be one-to-one, and it is unproblematic if what is strongly differentially explained is a function of arguments in several different explanatory conditions.

We need, though, to distinguish between two different kinds of recoverability. The first I will label *jump* recoverability. (In what follows, 'p' and 'q' are schematic for sentences with a specific time reference.) p is jump recoverable from q iff given all the initial conditions at some stage or other in the explanatory chain from p to q, other than p itself and conditions explained by p, and given also the covering law involved at each stage, and q itself, one can infer to the truth of p. There is jump recoverability of a statement of the pattern of colours in the original scene from a description of the picture produced by a normal camera. But there is also jump recoverability in cases that were not intuitively examples of differential explanation. There is jump recoverability in the second camera case: for one can infer that unless the colours were a certain way in the original scene, no picture would have been taken at all, and one has the information that a picture was produced.

The concept we need in explaining strong differential explanation is not jump recoverability, but rather *stepwise* recoverability. We have stepwise recoverability of p from q iff in the explanatory chain from p to q, at each stage, given just the initial conditions of that stage other than the explanandum of the previous stage, and given also the explanandum of the present stage and its covering law, one can recover the explanandum of the previous stage. There is not stepwise recoverability in the second camera example because at the stage at which what is to be explained is a statement of the distribution of the shades of grey on the film, we cannot recover the pattern of colours that light had just from the effect on the film and a knowledge of how the light affects the film. It is at this stage that there is, intuitively, a loss of sensitivity, and the definition of stepwise recoverability captures this intuition. So jump recoverability does not imply stepwise recoverability; in fact another counterexample would be provided by our DNA example.

Does the introduction of stepwise recoverability make the other part of the account of DE, the notion we earlier explained of weak DE, redundant? It seems that it does not, for there are examples in which we have stepwise recoverability without weak DE, and they are intuitively cases of deviant causal chains. For example, a quite specific type of retinal image might trigger an unstructured signal which in turn stimulates a memory image which causes an experience similar to the image. We can fill out this example in such a way that there is stepwise recoverability, but not weak DE. So both conditions seem to be needed, since (according to my intuitions) it would not be an example of perception.

There are several questions that may be raised about stepwise recoverability.[18] How much information are we allowed to lose at each stage of the explanatory chain, consistent with stepwise recoverability? For surely *some* will be lost at each stage in any chain. And how detailed a statement are we given, when we are required to recover from it a certain explanans sentence? The answer to the first of these two questions seems to be that the degree of detail that must be preserved is determined by the description relative to which the chain is being assessed as deviant or not. Roughly speaking, we may say that if we are concerned with whether an experience as of its being ϕ is perceptual under that description, then we must be able to stepwise recover that it really *is* ϕ from the information given when we apply the definition of stepwise recoverability to the example. Thus if an experience is to be perceptual under the description 'as of there being a source of light in front of one', it is not necessary to recover nearly so detailed a statement as is required if the experience is to be perceptual under the description 'as of a Victorian gas lamp in front of one in a light mist'.

[18] Some of those that follow were raised by Paul Benaceraff and Saul Kripke.

An answer to the second question would presumably also involve a relativity. When the issue is whether someone ϕ'd intentionally, the statement from which recovery is to be made will be as general a description of the agent's bodily movement as is consistent with a movement so described being a bodily movement of the kind the putative agent believes to be a ϕ-ing in the circumstances in which he believes himself to be. It would not be a description of the precise path in space traced by his limbs. In the two cases not so far mentioned, those of explanation of an experience and of explanation by an intention, we would need to supplement the information given according to the definition of stepwise recoverability with statements about which neurophysiological states, for the perceiver or agent at the time, realize his having that experience or intention. (There is more on this notion of realization in Chapter III, section 1.) In the perception case, for the experience to be a perception as of its being ϕ, one would require stepwise recoverability of its being ϕ from a statement of the person's neurophysiological condition that for him realizes his having then an experience as of its being ϕ. Conversely, in the action case, for intentionality under the description ϕ of a bodily movement, one would require stepwise recoverability of the neurophysiological condition which in fact for him then realizes his possessing the intention to ϕ from a description (of the kind we discussed) of that movement.

The way I have answered these questions leaves room for the following possibility. On one occasion when throwing darts I may intend to hit the bulls' eye; a few moments later I may intend to hit a point half a centimetre to the right of the bull's-eye. In so far as I have beliefs about the bodily movements which will in each case produce my goal, and given my high degree of incompetence at darts, it may well be true that they are not in fact distinct types of bodily movement which I believe are going to produce the two distinct results. Is what I have said consistent with this evident possibility?

I would say that in the two cases there is *a* sense in which I have the same intention in each case: the first time I intend to hit the bull's-eye in making a movement of a certain kind, and a few moments later I intend to hit a point half a centimetre to the right of it in making a movement of that same kind. How is it that I am not inconsistent? This is really not such an unfamiliar situation. It is a case of a relational belief of a movement-type M: I believe of M that it has one property, and also of it that it has another, where these are properties that I know to be incompatible. But we know that Ralph has often been in such a relation to Bernard J. Ortcutt.[19] (There will no doubt be a number of explanations possible of how I fail to appreciate the identity of the bodily movement type in question: perhaps I confuse a different direction of squinting with a different type of movement.)

The linear restrictions implicit in the account of stepwise recoverability so far given can be dropped. For instance, it does not matter if there is a loss of sensitivity at some stage if what fails to differentially explain at that stage re-enters the explanatory network at a later stage via a different path. An example raised by Gilbert Harman can be used to illustrate the point. Suppose someone wants to take a photograph of a particular scene, and the only way he can do so in his circumstances is to build a camera like the second camera. Would we not want to say that a picture produced by this camera is a picture of both the shapes and the colours of the original scene? But is there not still a loss of sensitivity and failure of stepwise recoverability at the stage at which an image forms on the black and white film? The answer to both these questions is affirmative. Now in Harman's example, the principle of operation of the colour conversion device are caused, via the photographer's intentions, by the colours of the original scene. The account I have suggested should be adapted to cases in which we consider not just a linear chain of explanations, but a tree-like structure. (This could be made formally precise, with some tedium in exchange for little illumination.) In the revised account, what strongly differentially explains in action or perception may divide into several ultimate components. Thus in Harman's example, the distribution of light classified by shades of grey is recoverable from the picture produced; but the grey/colour associations of the original scene are also recoverable from the properties of the colour conversion device, and on the tree structure account, we can use the grey/colour associations of the original scene to recover fully the original scene. This would be allowed because the principle of operation of the colour conversion device are themselves explained, via the agent's intentions, by those associations. On such an account, the criterion of nondeviance would be both tree-like and recursive.

With so much by way of discussion of strong differential explanation behind us, let us return to the example of the memory cells. In particular, let us return to the position of someone who finds the studio examples we gave earlier plausible as counterexamples to the necessity of counterfactual theories, but when presented with the memory cell example finds it attractive to say that there fortuitously a perceptual mechanism is set up. The point I have to make here is that this person can still be satisfied with a noncounterfactual theory thus: we could impose for nondeviance of chain the requirement of stepwise recoverability, but without the condition that there be a function in the covering law of each stage of the kind we discussed earlier. Such a position will employ some notion of recoverability, but it would not amount to the kind of sensitivity we were concerned to elucidate: for instance, in the cell example, the signal that activates the content of any given memory cell may be quite unstructured, and so may not intuitively specifically reflect the original retinal image that caused it.

Such a position is not the one for which I have been arguing, but it does prompt a question about that latter position. We can imagine a kind of example like the previous one about the memory cells, but in which the triggering of the contents of the memory storage cells is done by structured signals that can indeed (by the function and stepwise recoverability conditions) be regarded as encoding details of the original scene. We can suppose that the signal operates as a key that opens the gate to the cell and allows activation of the image; suppose too that the 'key' is tried simultaneously at many different locks, and that in the diagram below, just the contents of cell 2 are stimulated, for instance because the signal has the unlocking type a2 for it. My intuitions are that not even this is an example of perception. *A fortiori* stepwise recoverability is fulfilled: for that held even when the signal was unstructured. And is there not also a function that is

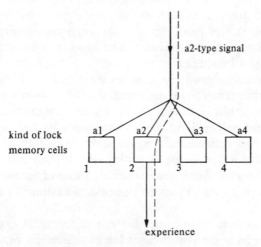

relevant? Given a knowledge of all the details of this mechanism, and of the final kind of experience produced, we can determine what external scene must have produced it; and such working out determines a function from the surrounding scene to the experience produced.

But it is not a function obtained in the right kind of way. I am concerned in strong differential explanation with functions referred to in the laws that cover links in the actual explanatory chain, the chain corresponding to the broken line in the diagram above. The properties of the cells unactivated on this occasion are irrelevant to whether there is such a function, and we should not consider their properties in examining whether the condition of strong differential explanation is met.

Here it may be helpful to recall the difference between two kinds of key. One sort is such that just one of a collection opens just one of a number of doors in a particular building. When such a key opens the door, the presence of a key of just that kind no more *differentially* explains the movement of the piece of metal previously locking the door than does the singular condition of the form *Fxt* when an explanation is covered by the very simple law we gave earlier. The signals that are keys in this latest version of the memory cell example are like this kind of key. The kind of key they would have to resemble to allow fulfilment of strong differential explanation would be more on the model of the plastic card that operates a machine at a bank: a pattern of dots on the card may strongly differentially explain the printing of your account number on the statement the machine delivers (but does not so explain the balance said to be there).

I have so far offered some considerations in favour of the view that fulfilment of the differential explanation condition is necessary for nondeviance of causal chain. I want now in both the action and perception cases to consider whether more needs to be added to differential explanation to obtain a sufficient condition of nondeviancy; in doing so, I shall also consider some rival theories of deviance, notably those of Strawson in the case of perception and Pears in the case of action.[20] Let us take action first.

One reason it may be thought that differential explanation ('DE') is not in general sufficient for nondeviance of chain is a feeling that one cannot simply 'walk into' an action aid, something that is in no way excluded by the requirement of DE. The thought seems to be that only after a certain amount of use of a mechanism can the bodily movements produced through it be intentional of the agent. (It can be the practice with the mechanism that matters to this objector, and not the absence of knowledge of how the mechanism works – this may still be absent after some practice.) But the principle that one cannot 'walk into' an action aid and start acting intentionally immediately does not seem to me to be acceptable. A doctor might help someone who suffers a deficiency disease preventing his neurons from transmitting messages, by getting him to take tablets that permit him to realize his intentions; the patient may start acting intentionally immediately. But a man with the same illness might accidentally happen to eat something containing the same substance, and then in realizing his intentions be acting intentionally. It is no answer to such an example to say that we can include this possibility just because the ingested substance restores a normal mechanism of working: for it need not – the substance consumed might be one not naturally found in the body, and its operation might involve bypassing (whilst fulfilling the DE condition) some of the usual

20 P. F. Strawson, 'Causation in Perception'; D. F. Pears, 'The Appropriate Causation of Intentional Basic Actions', *Critica* 7 (1975).

steps. Indeed in one famous actual example, the former condition was fulfilled.[21]

A second objection to the sufficiency of DE for nondeviancy is provided by the thought that the DE requirement does not exclude the possibility that the chain from intention to bodily movement pass through the intentions of a second person. This second person might for instance be a knowledgeable neurophysiologist who decides on a particular occasion to produce in me exactly the motor impulses needed to realize what he knows, from my neurophysiological states, to be my intentions. Is my bodily movement really intentional when my arm moves exactly as I intended it to? It is not plausible to say that it is so without qualification. Why is this so?

It may be said that it is so because it is not true in such an example that it is reliably the case that if there is a bodily movement of the (putative) agent, then it is one that matches his intention: the intervening neurophysiologist might not have chosen to produce the corresponding movement. But the absence of this kind of reliability, 'conditional reliability' as it is naturally called, cannot be the explanation of the deviancy. Conditional reliability in the absence of DE is not sufficient for nondeviancy, as the Chopin example (p. 56) shows, and in the presence of DE it is much too strong to require it for nondeviancy of chain. There could be a substance in the brain that is, for a given person, only fortuitously present, and which stops neural messages becoming scrambled: if this substance were absent, it could be reliably the case that some bodily movement were made, though there would in general then be no matching with the intention. So if the substance were not reliably present, a conditional reliability requirement would not be fulfilled. This would not prevent intentionality of the putative agent's bodily movements under appropriate descriptions when the substance did happen to be present.

[21] The case of L-DOPA: see Oliver Sacks's engrossing descriptions and history in his book *Awakenings* (London: Pelican, 1976). The substance in the relevant part of the brain is not L-DOPA, but dopamine: dopamine however cannot be absorbed by the brain (see Sacks, p. 54), and so L-DOPA was fed to the patients.

Note that such examples can be adapted to show that it is incorrect to require for the intentionality of a ϕ-ing under that description that the agent's belief that he *can* ϕ in the circumstances be knowledge: this would not be true in a drug example in which the agent has inferred from false premises that the drugs he is taking will restore a certain mechanism which they in fact bypass.

A better reason is provided by David Pears in his treatment of a somewhat similar example.[22] Of the concept of the originator of an action, he writes that 'the description of [such examples] naturally puts a great strain on such a conservative concept'. When we say that an event is, under a given description, intentional of a person, we normally imply that that person was the originator of that event. It is not clear whether there is such a person as *the* originator of the bodily movement in our example, but if there is, it is certainly not the person whose brain the neurophysiologist is inspecting. If the implication about origination is to be retained, then the requirement of DE must be filled out to one that also requires that the chain from intention to bodily movement should not run through the intentions of another person.[23]

One consideration that might make someone reluctant to accept such a modified DE account as sufficient for nondeviancy is this. If a man fortuitously comes to be equipped with an action aid, then from his point of view it may well be a matter of luck that his psychological states produce matching actions: but this is hardly our normal picture of intentional action. It is hard to state this objection without supplying an answer to it. A plausible case may be made that the intention to ϕ implies the belief that one will ϕ;[24] so if the appropriate belief is absent, so will the intention be. But there is also another point to be made about such cases. It is not obvious that an event of ϕ-ing can be said to be intentional under that description only if the agent intended to ϕ. If a man acts in the hope of success, while believing his chances to be infinitesimal, but thinking he has nothing to lose by trying, then we may be reluctant to make so strong a statement as that he intends to bring about the event under the given description (we can say only that he is aiming

[22] 'The Appropriate Causation of Intentional Basic Actions', p. 66.

[23] Clearly some obvious refinements are appropriate here. For instance, if I suffer from akinesia, and I get another person to move my arm for me, and this movement is a signalling to a third person outside the window, it may not be wrong to say that the movement of my arm (*not* my moving it – no such thing occurred) is intentional under a description relating to signalling. If we decide it is, then the additional requirement of the text must be restricted to descriptions that are 'basic' in the agent's plan.

[24] For answers to some possible objections to this claim, see Paul Grice's 'Intention and Uncertainty' (British Academy Lecture, 1971), pp. 4–5; and also Harman, 'Practical Reasoning', *Review of Metaphysics* 29 (1976).

at it); but it would be wrong apparently to say in a case in which he succeeds that the event produced was not intentional of him. In such examples, one may even be quite ignorant of how the desired consequence will come about if indeed it does come about.[25]

3. COMPARISONS WITH RIVAL THEORIES

I fear that the view I have so far defended about the conditions for nondeviancy in the action case makes me, in the terminology of David Pears, a 'psychological feudalist': 'although [psychological feudalism] allows that some physiological infrastructure is needed, it treats the nature and work of the actual serfs as wholly irrelevant to life at the top.'[26] Pears himself has a different theory of deviance, and towards the end of a fascinating paper he himself gives this summary of the restrictions he would suggest in order to exclude the deviant chains from intention to bodily movement.

First, the agent must intend to bring about the bodily movement through the essential initiating event. Second, he must intend that the sequence of intermediate stages that follow that event should belong to a reliable type. Third, the reliable type of sequence must be specified in his intention as either the normal type for human agents or else a variation produced by a prosthetic device which is, in some sense, part of himself and operated by himself alone.[27]

The 'essential initiating event' takes place in the cortex, but nevertheless according to Pears the first condition above does not require all (or even any) human agents to have knowledge of events under neurophysiological descriptions. For my given intention to produce a bodily movement, the corresponding event (if such exists) has a psychological description: 'it is the act of will to make that particular movement' (p. 65).

[25] Nevertheless, at this point, I have much less confidence in the sufficiency of the DE account than in its necessity. There is some discussion of what we might need to add to reach sufficiency in section 4 of this chapter.
[26] 'The Appropriate Causation of Intentional Basic Actions', p. 56. I should perhaps say explicitly that I do not hold the findings of the physiological sciences to be irrelevant to the *extension* of the physiological concepts in question, but only to the concepts themselves.
[27] Ibid., p. 68. I should in fairness note that David Pears has told me that he no longer places any weight on reliability in excluding deviant chains.

These initiating events are the causal basis of the agent's noninferential (fallible) knowledge that he is making what he takes to be the appropriate movement. Now perhaps a clever neurophysiologist might succeed in severing the causal route from such initiating events back to the agent's beliefs. But even if that did prove to be possible, that would clearly not be any objection to Pears's view: even if such initiating events might not then be properly described as 'acts of will', they are still of the same physiological kind in important respects as those that were, and this could be said to be part of what is distinctive of nondeviant chains. Nor is it obviously an objection that the account works only for humans, and not for all conceivable rational agents: for an act of will may with a degree of plausibility be identified with an event of trying, and a case may perhaps be made[28] that such events are required conceptually for intentional action, that is, in nondeviant chains in this field.

The difficulty for Pears's suggestion lies rather in the possibility of deviance in the chain after an appropriate initiating event: the kind of case that would arise if, for instance, a neurophysiologist connected up certain parts of a man's central nervous system in such a way that after occurrences of a given kind of initiating event, the resulting impulse travels along the artificially produced path and causes nervousness. Pears holds that nervousness imports deviance because 'nervousness is not a reliable type of link in the sequence of stages leading to [action of the intended type]' (op. cit., p. 68). I will consider reliability below. But we can note now that it cannot be the complete story, because there are cases where the chain is completely reliable after an appropriate initiating event, but in which the bodily movement is not intentional under the appropriate description – for instance, it might well be that Chopin and anyone with a similar history simply could not intend to play the piano as if nervous, attempt to act on this intention, and also succeed in producing a bodily movement intentional under not only the description 'playing the piano' but also under the description 'as if nervous'. (Of course, the nervous-

---

[28] For a colourful defence of such a view, a defence that contains additional material that need not be adopted by someone who holds the view in question, see Brian O'Shaughnessy, 'Trying (as the Mental "Pineal Gland")', *Journal of Philosophy* 70 (1973): 365–86.

ness could be accommodated in Chopin's plan; but this would be like the imagined servant of Freud we considered earlier, and is not a feature of the case now in question.) We still need the requirement of differential explanation to exclude this kind of example: reliability is not sufficient.

David Pears's first two conditions start 'the agent intends that . . .'. This seems to require that any human agent have particular propositional attitudes with respect to acts of will or events of trying if he is to ct intentionally; and this does not seem to be necessary: hov ever necessary such events may be for intentional action, it dues not seem to be necessary that the agent have any particular attitudes with respect to those events. A defender of Pears on this point might try to appeal to 'the' causal theory of perception: it is still true, he may say, that a man's experience is a perception of a given object only if a certain kind of causal connection links the object with the man, whether he believes the causal theory of perception or not. This is of course quite true, but it does not parallel Pears's claim on intentional action because in the perceptual case we require only connections of a certain kind (partly given in the differential explanation condition) and not belief in or other attitudes about those connections.

What of reliability? We saw that Pears required that the sequence of intermediate stages from the initiating event 'belong to a reliable type'. We need to be very careful here. On the one hand, as we saw, some kinds of reliability seem not to be sufficient: there might be some kinds of action or even kinds of bodily movement such that it is a nomologically true generalization for creatures of the species in question that any-one intending to perform an action or movement of that kind under certain conditions will act out of nervousness.[29] On the

---

[29] There is a puzzling passage about reliability in Pears's paper (p. 67): I will quote five consecutive sentences from it:

'If the motor nerves to my left hand were almost gone, I would seldom succeed in clenching it. But when I did clench it, I would be doing so intentionally. Such examples could be multiplied. They show that it is too much to require that the prior stages of a basic action should be reliable. All that we ought to require is that they should belong to a reliable type of sequence.'

Why does the clenching example meet this last requirement? This is to ask what the verifying reliable type of sequence might be in the example. It cannot be that specified by 'chain beginning with an initiating event (act of will) continuing with an impulse through the remaining nerves', for that is not reliable. Is the case

other hand, some kinds of reliability appear not to be necessary. For instance a quite nondeviant ordinary chain meeting the differential explanation condition may have a stage that produces the next stage with a probability of only 10 per cent: this seems to me not to cast doubt on the intentionality of the resulting movement in cases where all the stages are so produced. Here to speak of a reliable *type* does not by itself save the requirement, for the type is not reliable.

These observations would still be compatible with the different requirement for nondeviancy of chain, that the circumstances that produce the sensitivity of the stages of an actual chain be reliably present when one is produced. So should we impose that? There are several considerations against doing so. First, the condition seems intuitively too strong. For instance, a man might be like the rest of us except that his brain cells do not reliably produce one of the substances required for the transmission of neural impulses: this fact seems to cast no doubt on the status of causal chains from intention to action when the substance is adequately produced upon a particular occasion. Similar observations apply if atmospheric conditions affect the operation of the prosthetic radio device we imagined earlier. Second, the condition is more clearly wrong in the perceptual case – for otherwise we would not be able to say that on a moonless night one could see an unlit farmhouse suddenly in a flash of lightning. Third, 'is nondeviant' is an absolute predicate of particular chains, and not at all relative to some further description or predicate; whereas 'reliably' is quite plausibly so relative. (Given that a child has spots of a certain kind, it's reliably measles; given he or she was born at c_1 or . . . or c_k, where the c_i are the birthplace coordinates of all those who get measles, it is not reliable.) Are the circumstances to be counted as reliably present absolutely, if they are reliably present under *some* description? Then it seems they will almost

---

one of intentional action because if such a chain operated and the other nerves were functional, then there would reliably be the effect of the required kind? But to allow that would trivialize the requirement, because any chain at all could be embedded in some circumstances or other that act as a failsafe mechanism. (We could not make use of the fact that in the clenching example, the additional circumstances are more of the same kind as those already present – more nerves – because we do not want to exclude the possibility of diverse kinds of efferent pathways in intentional action for some conceivable creatures.)

always count as reliably present (with the approximate truth of physical determinism on the macroscale). But the circumstances will never count as reliably present if required to be so relative to *every* description of those circumstances.[30]

It is of course not enough simply to argue against the reliability condition: we must also treat the examples others have invoked the reliability condition to explain. One vivid case is given by Pears[31] who discusses a gunman who intends to fire his gun and whose cortex sends out the initiating event: unknown to the gunman, the nerve to his index finger has been severed, but the intended movement still takes place because the impulse produced by the initiating event attracts some lightning which itself generates the required impulse in the severed section of the nerve. Pears says there is a strong case against calling the firing of the gun intentional because the performance lacks primary reliability, that is, the goal was not 'achieved by dependable stages'.[32] However, the probability case suggests that dependability is not required, and the example of the prosthetic radio device can easily be modified so that it is something external that is not dependably present and produces a nondeviant chain.

Does this mean the criterion of differential explanation commits us to saying Pears's gunman acts intentionally? No: on that criterion, the judgement has to turn on further details of the case. If the mechanism by which the impulse attracts the lightning is (roughly) such that, in the actual circumstances, it could easily have attracted lightning that would have produced impulses with quite different effects, the condition on specific reflection will fail and the movement will not be intentional – the differential explanation of the movement under the description 'movement of a kind believed in the circumstances to be a squeezing of a trigger' will relate not to the properties of the impulse but to the properties of the lightning present (where these are not in turn differentially explained by properties of the impulse). On the other hand, if there is specific reflection, the lightning is no different from a rather

---

[30] A fourth problem might be that a definition employing reliability might wrongly make the intentionality of a particular action intrinsically a matter of degree.

[31] 'The Appropriate Causation of Intentional Basic Actions', p. 59.

[32] Ibid., p. 52.

unreliable external action aid, of a kind a patient might think at least better than nothing.[33]

It may be felt that it does not matter whether the agent's bodily movement specifically reflects the gunman's intention or not: the movement is not intentional in either case when lightning so forms part of the causal chain. One source of this intuition may be that the gunman may not have had the slightest reason to believe that the lightning would ever occur. But then our man who happened to eat food containing L-DOPA may not have had the slightest reason to believe that he would consume any of the substance either, yet he acted intentionally. Perhaps then the point is that the agent must not have a false belief, such as that if there is any lightning it will not help him? But then our man may have false beliefs about his internal neurophysiology, and believe falsely that if there is any L-DOPA in his food, that will not help him perform the bodily movement. I am tentatively inclined to think that we should say that, in the lightning example, when there is specific reflection of the agent's intention, principles suggested by other examples lend support to the view that the movement is intentional. But I do so with unease.

There is a version of the reliability requirement that is not touched by these criticisms. A nondeviant chain, it may be said, need not be such that it is reliably the case that: if a chain of its kind is given an input (the intention to ϕ/its being ϕ at a certain place), it delivers a matching output (an action believed to be a ϕ-ing/an experience as of its being ϕ). Rather what is required is: it is reliably the case that *if* a chain of that kind is given an input *and* it in fact delivers an output, the output will match the input in the sense required for the given scheme of holistic explanation. But this is precisely the requirement of 'conditional reliability' we considered and rejected several pages ago. We may also note the following point in addition to the arguments that were given then. There is a

---

[33] I should emphasize that I am not here committing myself to the need for a reliability requirement outside what Pears characteristically calls the 'vestibule' of action (op. cit.), that is, in the stages of the chain later than those from the intention to the bodily movement: in fact I am sceptical of the correctness of either a primary reliability requirement or the need for match with the stages envisioned in the agent's plan outside the vestibule.

sense in which, subsequent to the initial 'accident', a perceptual system may meet a requirement of conditional (or stronger) reliability if it has a triggering device analogous to the one opening the second shutter in our second camera example, delivering on to the retina of the system the contents of some memory store. We do seem to need the refinement that differential explanation supplies, or at least the features this idea attempts to capture.[34]

Now let us consider another rival theory, that of Strawson,[35] which it may be claimed offers a better account of the examples we have already cited in the case of perception.

Strawson agrees with Grice that for an experience to be the perception it seems that a certain causal connection is required between what it seems to be of and the experience itself; and he agrees also that this condition is not sufficient. But the extra that is required for a sufficient condition is not, according to him, to be gained by placing further restrictions upon the mode of causal dependence: rather, the counterexamples such as the brain case and Kinglake's hallucination are to be excluded by certain restrictions implicit in the naïve concept of perception. These restrictions flow from and are unified by the idea of a spatiotemporal location of an observer and his perspective or point of view at that location with that oreintation. Thus one can see only what is not masked or obstructed from one; one can see only what is in a certain spatial range, one's arc of vision, and so forth. The hallucinating man does not count as perceiving his own brain because that is mased from him by his cranium; Kinglake did not really hear the bells because of the remoteness of that event from him in time at the time of his experience. Strawson holds that as knowledge of perceptual mechanisms increases, it is natural to introduce superior, refined concepts of perception and these will very likely make reference to *kinds* of causal dependence; but, he holds, we should recognize these developments as just that, refinements of the naïve concept, rather than as verdicts. of a pretheoretical

---

[34] It should be noted too that the 'reliably *matching*' interpretation of the reliability condition would count as nondeviant the causal chain in the gunman and lightning case in the version in which there *is* 'specific reflection'.

[35] 'Causation in Perception'. Page references are to the version in *Freedom and Resentment and Other Essays*.

concept on newly discovered actual examples. It should be clear that the criterion of differential explanation I have proposed places me in disagreement with Strawson's position, and I should in fairness note before developing the point further that Strawson himself is extremely tentative in stating his own view: '*perhaps* the point is a fine one, *perhaps* not ultimately settleable', he writes (p. 81).

We may note in passing that Strawson's account of the perceptual case is prima facie not generalizable to the action case, with which we have seen so many parallels: for his solution makes reference to the idea of a spatiotemporal point of view which (apparently) has no analogue in the explanation of intentional action. But of course this remark should not prevent consideration of Strawson's theory in its own right. (Perhaps this hope of a unified account is merely a chimaera produced by an over-ambitious theory.)

A second preliminary observation to be made before we consider the details of Strawson's account is that there is one important respect in which an account employing differential explanation sides with him and against some more extreme conceivable views. Strawson holds (in his own words, my italics), 'it does not seem that there is any concealed, implicit reference, *however unspecific*, to modes or mechanisms of causal dependence' in the naïve concept of perception (p. 81). The DE account differs from this in placing restrictions on the kind of dependence. But on the other hand, the DE condition sides *with* Strawson in that the restrictions it imposes on the causal chain are not stated in concepts drawn from the special sciences, concepts unavailable to the everyday master of the naïve concept of perception. So the view I am defending is less extreme than one according to which the results of scientific investigation are relevant to a correct specification of the *concept* of a perceptual experience (or an intentional action).[36]

---

[36] 'But you yourself use technical concepts from the philosophy of explanation in elucidating differential explanation.' But there are expressions in ordinary use whose mastery requires some tacit grasp of the concept of DE, a concept that of course does not need to be introduced via any particular *a posteriori* science. For example, we have already noted that 'explains' is undoubtedly sometimes used in the sense of 'differentially explains' (as when someone insists that in the second camera example, what explains the distribution of colours in the picture is not the distribution of colours in the external scene). An example of a concept that perhaps embeds the notion of DE is that of a *fossil*.

In discussing Strawson's account I shall be aiming to establish the following case: that where Strawson's restrictions diverge from the account I have suggested, the verdicts given by the (or at least my) naïve concept of perception are predicted by the account appealing to DE; that where the Strawsonian restrictions are read without any limitation on the mode of causal dependence, there is a serious threat of circularity; and that where Strawson's principles are correct, an essential element in their correctness is the application of some concept in conformity with the DE account. These three claims may be illustrated as follows:

(i) Strawson's explanation of the hallucinating brain example is that this is no case of perception because the brain is masked from the putative perceiver by the (opaque) cranium. But this explanation does not cover all the cases on which the naïve concept confidently pronounces: for if our crania were transparent, and our heads of such a shape that one could normally see a corner of one's brain through it, and a hallucinating man had an experience as of such a corner of his brain, it seems clear (and on the basis of the naïve concept) that this would not *ipso facto* make the case into one of perception. Strawson defends the claim that *some* causal requirement is implicit in the naïve concept of perception on the ground that Lady Macbeth's waiting gentlewoman will realize that she cannot cure her lady's hallucination by spreading some actual blood on her hands; and equally we may say that when someone is hallucinating an experience as of some corner of his brain as a result of taking a drug, we need no refinement of the concept of perception in order to understand the idea that his hallucination is not removed or turned into a perception by replacing part of his cranium with a newly shaped and transparent component. It seems to me that this point, if taken, shows that restrictions on the external positioning of the perceiver together with general requirements on causation and matching will never be sufficient to capture the naïve concept of perception: be they ever so difficult to state within the acceptable constraints of a philosophical analysis, the naïve concept still does impose restrictions upon the internal stage of the causal chain.

It may be said that Strawson could meet the case of the hallucinating transparent cranium by naturally extending his theory thus. Once we have a set of conditions, such as his 'restrictions', any one of which may block perception, they may be naturally extended to a wider set by the following principle: if a person has an experience, and none of the restriction conditions is violated, the experience may nevertheless fail to count as perception if it is true that if one of them *were* to be violated in the circumstances, the experience would still be present. This would then exclude the case of the transparent cranium because if an opaque object obstructed the relevant (part of the) cranium from the experiencer, there would still be an experience of the given kind there actually is.[37] However my point (ii) is that Strawson cannot legitimately use the obstruction restrictions, and I turn immediately to this.

(ii) Strawson appealed to facts about obstruction to block some putative counterexamples to his account. But of course spatial obstruction does not hinder sight if the obstructing object is transparent (otherwise glasses could never aid vision and one could never see someone through a window). Now what are transparent objects? They are ones that are not merely translucent, they are ones you can *see* through. So to limit Strawson's restriction to nontransparent objects would be circular. Appeal might in principle be made to relative non-distortion of the light pattern as a definition of transparency: but to do so would reintroduce reference to modes of causal dependence which Strawson seemed to wish to avoid.[38] Strawson's view that there is no such restriction 'however unspecific' seems to block even attempts to explain transparency in terms that appeal to the normal mode of transmission and not the concept of light as such.

(iii) My third comment is on the implicit use of DE and other considerations in the application of some of the concepts

[37] Note, though, that this extension of Strawson's theory would have to be modified to accommodate the possibility that if a condition that violated one of the restrictions were to obtain, it might be one that itself caused a previously perceptual experience to be hallucinatory.

[38] I am thus not in agreement with Pears who writes it is 'only Strawson's treatment of the internal stage' of the causal chain that is vulnerable to objections (see 'The Causal Conditions of Perception', *Synthèse* 33 (1976): 36).

In fact it is not at all obvious that Strawson's obstruction restrictions are true even when applied only to opaque objects. Light rays are bent by large objects like the sun in a way that may allow an observer on earth to see a star that is in (*some*) spatial sense obstructed from him by another heavenly body.

used in the restrictive principles to which Strawson appeals and which he says flow from the idea of a spatio-temporal point of view. Consider the notion of the 'arc of vision' (p. 79). An arc of vision for a perceiver with a given oreintation at a given point (with a given location for other objects) is a volume of space, for it is that within which an object must lie to be visible by that perceiver then. But it is clear that regions of space that correspond with the perceiver's 'blind spot' must be excluded, even though neither masked nor obstructed: for objects in that region are not counted as visible by that perceiver then, even if (by techniques now familiar from the previous examples) these objects play a causal role in the production of an experience. (More spectacular cases may be constructed if we imagine the perceiver to be suffering from scotoma, an obscuration of part of the visual field.) Another example concerns the *range* of a given sense, a concept also employed by Strawson. It seems plain that the range of a sense not only varies with the occasion and (in the case of human sight), say, the conditions of illumination; but also on a given occasion with the conditions of illumination in various regions of a volume of space. A man on board a yacht sailing parallel to the resorts on the Côte d'Azur at night may be able to see what happens on the front at Cannes and not what is happening on the surface of the water between him and the town. What unifies the visible regions on an occasion and from occasion to occasion? My claim is that it is in part the sensitivity of the stages of chains from the objects within these regions to the experiences, which is in these examples the ground of differential explanation. Of course the *a posteriori* ground of such sensitivity is the reflection of light from these regions (or objects in these regions); but it is not necessary for the position developed here to maintain that the concept of light, that physical phenomenon, enters the naïve concept of perception; what matters is the resulting differential explanation itself, which has been defined without reference to any particular physical phenomenon.

4. REFINEMENTS

What is the role of examples in fixing the extension of 'perceives'? There can be no objection of general principle to the view that the extension is fixed in part by citing particular sequences of objects that stand in this relation. Such a procedure need not be circular if the examples are not specified (as they need not be) using 'perceives' or expressions to be defined in terms of it. Just such a general picture of the fixing of the extension of natural kind terms has rightly come to seem plausible from the work of Kripke and Putnam, and the arguments used in defence of that picture might be applied too in the case of perception. It is of no avail to argue that either the examples used in fixing the extension of perception have some common property in virtue of which they are all instances of perception (so we could just state the common property and omit the examples), or else they do not and the extension has not properly been unified. For such an alleged dilemma ignores the now familiar possibility that the unifying principle supplied by the examples can classify together the objects in the extension and yet be discovered *a posteriori* from the examples: again, compare gold and its atomic structure.

Nevertheless, this said, there seem to be strong reasons for not applying the natural kind model to the determination of the extension of 'perceives'. In the case of gold, we are confident that a few samples (indeed one) will fix the extension of 'gold' (given that it is a substance-word), because we are confident that there are scientifically fundamental characteristics from which the other relevant properties of the samples flow. But in the case of perception, even if we could give, as we could well hope to, an account of what scientifically identified relations underlie and explain some identified actual examples of the relation of perception, that would not properly fix the extension of 'perceives'. To mention a few reasons: we wish to apply the concept of perception to conceivable creatures with different physico-chemical realizations from our own; we wish to allow prosthetic devices and re-routings in internal stages of the chain at the very least; and so forth. The concept of perception, unlike that of a substance, is not one which determines a notion of kind such that any example of perception falls under a unique kind, and such that what is quite generally necessary and sufficient for perception can be discovered by empirical investigation of examples of that kind. Thus we cannot wholly avoid the traditional hard work of the method of imagined examples and the testing against them of the appropriate intuitions of those who have mastered the concept of perception.[39]

Does this show that the mention of particular instances of the perception relation does not have any role to play in fixing the extension of 'perceives'? I do not think so, for it is plausible to say that there is a different role that has to be played by it. This is the identification of *which* stage of a nondeviant, sensitive chain is the one such that objects at that stage are said to be the objects perceived. In an adequately sensitive chain, a full analysis would need to filter out perfectly differentially explanatory stages both earlier and later than the desired ones. Among sensitive later stages to be excluded are electro-chemical cross-sections of the optic nerve, the pattern of light in the lens of the eye, and so forth. We have an earlier stage that needs to be excluded if the perceptible state of a perceived object specifically reflects its state five minutes ago; or again a man might make an object whose perceptible qualities are geared by radio transmission to the perceptible qualities of some qualitatively identical object outside the range of any of a perceiver's senses, so that the condition of differential explanation of the man's experiences is met under suitable conditions by the wrong object. It is plausible that the appropriate *stage*

[39] In 'The Causal Conditions of Perception' Pears writes of Strawson's objection to Grice that it is circular to say that the appropriate causal chains for perception are those of the kind(s) operative in normal cases of perception, and says that it

'goes too far. For Grice's account of the causal line appropriate to seeing implies that it is a single line, or, at least, a limited disjunction of lines, and this is certainly not something that guarantees its own truth in a circular way. It is a contingent fact . . . the general causal connection between objects and the visual experiences that match them might have followed a largely different line on each occasion. Although this is extremely improbable, it is not inconceivable' (p. 30).

Presumably Strawson could reply to one of the points Pears is making here by noting that a definition can be circular without it being true that anything not falling under it necessarily fails to fall under it. But there is also a threat to a simple Gricean position in Pears's further observations here, because even if there are only a few causal routes followed in actual cases of perception, the view that there could have been many imposes an obligation on those elucidating the concept of perception to state the condition in virtue of which those hypothetical routes would in the hypothetical circumstances be sufficient for perception. Pears's own later appeal (p. 33) to the reliable delivery of matching visual experiences suggests that the smallness of the number of actual routes is not playing an essential part in his defence of his views.

of a sensitive chain is fixed by examples.[40] In the case of human vision, it is an *a posteriori* fact that the objects thus fixed (in a further elaboration of the condition) are roughly those such that the specific pattern of light reaching the perceiver is caused by reflection of light off those objects' surfaces in the case of ambient light, or by emission from them in the case of radiant light.

There is a competing suggestion about the means of determination of the stage of the causal chain such that objects at that stage may be said to be perceived. We were eager to allow much earlier that the substituends for 'ϕ' in 'experience as of its being ϕ' may include physical object vocabulary: an experience may be as of a girl walking across Hyde Park at a certain time of year, as viewed from a particular angle. Why should not the fixing of the appropriate stage of the causal chain be done by the content of these descriptions? For they certainly speak of objects of a kind found at only a certain stage of the causal chain; and it need in no way be required for such a suggestion that all the objects of the kinds mentioned in the 'as of' description of a perceptual experience count as perceived. The suggestion might be an initial restriction upon which further supplementary conditions are imposed. Yet even with these points noted, there seem to be severe difficulties in developing the proposal. Even when the description of what the experience is as of includes physical object vocabulary, and is the one it is entirely natural for the perceiver to offer, and the experience *is* a perception, this proposal can pick out the wrong stage. For a man may from time to time have opaque bodies floating in the fluid of his eye or chemical patches on his retina and know from an oculist that this is the usual cause of experiences of a certain kind that he has: the description of his experience 'as of the opaque bodies in the fluid of my eyes

---

[40] If the relevant stage is so fixed, we would expect it to be indeterminate whether a person could in principle see by means of sound waves. And it does seem to be thus indeterminate. More generally, from the arguments I have already given we ought to expect a range of indeterminacy. I argued against applying the natural kind model to 'perceives' on the ground that there was no scientifically fundamental characteristic for examples to fix: and similar considerations apply to the right stage of the causal chain. I should add, though, that I do not at all mean to exclude the possibility of evolutionary explanations of why we fix the extension of 'perceives' as we do.

floating around again' (or 'as of the chemical patterns on my
retina again') may be the one he naturally offers. If on a
particular occasion this is a fair description of his experience,
and yet this once there *are* opaque bodies suspended in the air,
but not in the fluid of his eye, then on our normal concept of
perception he does count as perceiving the bodies in the air:
but on a simple version of the suggestion being considered, he
would not count as perceiving them, for they are not at the
stage of the eye in the causal chain. There would too of course
be problems about experiences that we want to count as
perceptions of an object and for which the experiencer can
offer only phenomenal descriptions. Presumably the defender of
this competing position will have to move to the view that the
appropriate stage of the chain is fixed by the following requirement: that it is the stage such that the (great?) majority of
descriptions of what experiences are 'as of', and that are cast
in physical object vocabulary, are in fact descriptions of objects
of a kind found at that stage. But this statement of the view
has the consequence that it is impossible, as a matter of the
nature of the concept of perception, that there should be a
community of people who, although they use the concept of
perception, and fix the same stage such that objects at that
stage are the candidates for perception as we ourselves do,
nevertheless have perceptual systems which are very much
more clogged than are ours, so that the great majority of their
'as of' descriptions in physical object vocabulary that are
applied to their experiences relate to misfunctionings in or
properties of their perceptual systems. Such a situation would
indeed be strange and unusual, and would have to meet other
conditions for the members of such a community to be able to
impose the structure needed if the minority of their experiences
that *are* of objects at the right stage is to be regardable as
produced by tracing a route in a spatio-temporal world; but
yet it seems quite implausible to say that all such cases are
conceptually excluded by the notion of perception. (For instance,
when there is misfunctioning or some blocking, the experiences produced might within the terms of a legitimate
example in fact, though of course not as an *a priori* necessity,
have distinctive phenomenal characteristics.) In any case, I
am not clear that the general suggestion being proposed is not

circular: for do we not say that our experiences are *as of* those states of affairs that involve objects that we ordinarily *perceive*?

There remain many examples which, although they meet the requirements both of differential explanation and the stage condition fixed by examples of the perception relation, yet their status as instances of perception may reasonably be questioned. They include cases of light from an object which is reflected off the surface by a mirror, hearing a voice over a telephone, or a gramophone record, watching television and, a rather different kind of case, that in which an intervening brain surgeon causes to be produced in me a visual experience that matches exactly what he himself is seeing. Even if we temporarily ignore that last kind of case, it would not be correct to say of the remaining cases that linguistic practice unambiguously delivers the verdict that they are cases of perception. One is said to see the car to the rear 'in the mirror', to have heard Schnabel 'on record', or the prime minister 'on the phone'. The fact that in answer to the question 'Which car did you see?' asked when one has seen one in the mirror, one cites a particular car as an appropriate answer, is not decisive in answering the question of whether there is unqualified perception in these examples. For the answer that specifies a particular car may be more appropriate not because perception here is unconditional, but because to say 'None at all' as one's answer is more misleading in that it would more usually be taken to imply that one had not seen a car even in the mirror.

The case of the experience-producing surgeon is rather different, because in the other examples it is not plausible to attribute their failure as unconditional examples of perception to a link between perception and knowledge: the qualifications 'in the mirror', 'on the phone', and so forth, are appropriate even when there is no question but that by being in such contact with the object the would-be perceiver is in a position to gain knowledge of the object. This is not in general so with the experience-producing surgeon: here it seems more attractive to explain the failure of unconditional perception by the failure of such a chain to be (in the relevant cases) a method of gaining knowledge of the objects that the surgeon himself perceives.

It would be too strong to state such a connection between

perception and knowledge like this: an experience is a perception of an object only if it is produced by a means that actually yields knowledge of that object. There are clear counter-examples to so tight a link. A man may know he is taking part in a series of experiments on perception and cortical stimulation; and he may have no idea of whether his current visual experience, as of a machine with dials on it, is a perception or not; but if this *is* an experience caused in the usual way by light reflected off the object reaching his eye, followed by the usual steps of the causal chain, the experiencer is seeing that machine with dials even though he is not thereby in a position actually to know that any such machine exists.[41] But of course this obvious kind of example in no way discredits a view according to which there is perception in these examples because the experience is produced by a means which in ordinary circumstances does yield knowledge of the putatively perceived object.

If there is such a link between perception and knowledge, then an additional requirement (and one that naturally covers our most recently introduced batch of examples) is that the experience, to be a perception, must be produced by the usual causal means (say a pattern of light) which is then processed by an operation sufficient in normal circumstances to yield, for the person whose experience it is, knowledge of those objects. The brain of the experience-producing surgeon will not always be such a processing mechanism; but when it is in the case of a particular surgeon, our judgement that the experience is perception goes in step with our judgement that beliefs caused by the experience may be knowledge.[42]

For anyone pursuing for their own sake the philosophy of perception and knowledge there are several questions to be investigated at this point, notably that of whether these

---

[41] For an outline of a theory of knowledge that handles the absence of knowledge in this example very satisfactorily, see Alvin Goldman, 'Discrimination and Perceptual Knowledge', *Journal of Philosophy* 73 (1976): 771–91.

[42] A requirement stated in terms of knowledge also suggests a fallback position if it turns out that there are examples in which nervousness plays a role in the production of an action, the nervousness does not enter the agent's plan, and where we cannot say that the agent was helped in performing an action by the nervousness. For nervousness is not part of a mechanism that produces (non-inferential) knowledge of one's future behaviour.

restrictions in terms of knowledge are too strong, whether they are themselves sufficient to exclude all the examples that we want to in which the causal chain goes through the will of another, or whether an independent requirement needs to be tacked on, and so forth. I shall not pursue these questions here because it is clear that any satisfactory consideration of them would involve a much more extensive enquiry into the theory of knowledge than is appropriate when our main concern is with holistic explanation and its structure. But it should be explicitly noted that an introduction of a link with knowledge in no way makes the role of differential explanation redundant: for there seem to be no examples in which we have a non-deviant chain but do not have strong differential explanation.

A connection with knowledge would explain why counterfactual theories are so close to the truth. Counterfactual sensitivity can be seen as derivative from differential explanation together with such a condition about mechanisms suitable for the production of knowledge. If something is a knowledge-acquisition device, then for a range of different circumstances its states will be differentially explained by those circumstances if they obtain. So we would expect in general a corresponding range of counterfactuals to hold, as long as the mechanism is not inhibited.

If the differential explanation theorist can appeal to knowledge-producing mechanisms, why could not the counterfactual theorist do so too? Thus the counterfactual theorist might say that he could then accommodate the studio example since there a standard knowledge-producing mechanism is operative, whereas in the redwood examples, none such is operative. But in fact we do not really have symmetry between the differential explanation and the counterfactual theories: the DE theorist can say that it is plausible that there are no cases of nondeviance in which we do not have differential explanation, while the counterfactual theorist cannot say there are no such cases which do not display counterfactual sensitivity. The threat is that the knowledge requirement is doing all the work for him.

It will have been clear when I have been discussing perception that I have been sliding between various locutions, and hiding a cluster of important smaller issues. I have written about the question of what makes an experience as of its being ϕ into a perception that it is ϕ. But plainly 'perceives that it is ϕ' is not a locution that will do just the work required of it, since it seems to imply that the perceiver believes that it's ϕ; whereas the question of belief should be left open by that of perception. The idea of the experience as of its being ϕ being a perception *tout court* is conversely too weak; this would be the case if I had an experience as of a green book on the table in front of me and yet the book was not green, or some stage in the relevant causal chain was not sensitive in the right way to its being green. There is no objection, however, to introducing a notion of an experience (a token event) e being perceptual under description D, somewhat analogously to the concept of a bodily movement (a token event) e being intentional under a description D. There are differences of course: for instance on one way of using the phrase 'intentional under description D', an event can be intentional under a description only if the event itself satisfies the description, while there is clearly no corresponding way of using 'perceptual under a description', for the descriptions in the perceptual case are what the experience is 'as of'. But it is fair to point out that we would already expect some asymmetry here between the perceptual and the action cases since the *a priori* principles of the spatial scheme have in their consequent (see section I.2 above) an 'as of' where the action ones do not: the action ones have as consequent 'then x (the agent) does what he takes to be a ϕ-ing', which of course may *be* a ϕ-ing, while the perceptual/spatial ones have 'then x (the perceiver) has an experience as of its being ϕ'.

Why is it that we do not in fact employ a notion of an experience being perceptual under a description? Well, what we *do* employ is the concept of perceiving an object; and presumably the empirical reason we normally find this sufficient to our purposes is that human beings' perceptual systems are so similar that in normal circumstances when we know roughly the environment in which x is placed and know what y is like, we know roughly the kind of experience the perceiver x will have given just the further information that x is perceiving y. Clearly no corresponding *a posteriori* truth holds with respect to the concept that we might introduce, viz. that of having an intention with respect to an object: 'An intention to do *what* with it?' is a reasonable question about an agent and an object even in normal circumstances.

I have not yet suggested a definition of the relation of perceiving an object, but there is a natural starting-point of some plausibility in the framework I have been offering. It is this:

An experience (token event) e is a perception of object x iff there is some property ψ such that
  (i) $\psi(x)$
  (ii) $\psi(x)$ is the differential explanation of e being an experience as of an object being ψ (at the time, for the possessor of the experience)
  (iii) $\psi(x)$ is a condition at the right stage of the causal chain as determined by the examples of 'perceives' used in fixing the concept.[43]

Thus suppose I have an experience as of a black speck of a certain shape on my spectacles. I may in fact really be seeing a ship just coming over the horizon, and if I am, on this definition I will count as seeing the ship because the differential explanation, at the appropriate stage of the chain, of my having an experience of just this kind is that the ship on the horizon is of a certain shape and made of an opaque substance. But I do not perceive the door of the bridge of the ship according to this definition, because there is nothing in an 'as of' clause describing the experience that is differentially explained by the door of the bridge of the ship being thus-and-so. I offer this definition as a first step in need of further elaboration.

The notions of perception and of intentional action are everyday ones and as such it is reasonable to require any

[43] Two comments on this definition: (a) The quantification into the 'differentially explains' context here is done consciously. I cannot answer the alleged objections to this here, except to say that 'explains' and 'differentially explains' are not transparent in the extremely strong sense (with respect to descriptions having narrower scope than the operators in question) required for the conditions of application for the Frege argument to be fulfilled. (b) The use of 'as of' does not produce circularity. e is an experience as of its being ϕ for person y at time t iff e is of the same phenomenal kind as an experience of y's that would be differentially explained by its being ϕ given y's physiological constitution at t and the environmental conditions at t. This explanation does not employ the concept of perception.

elucidation of them to have an adequate answer to the question
'What is the *point* of the distinction?', in particular here, the
distinction between deviant and nondeviant chains. Further, an
adequate answer to this question should appeal to and not go
beyond everyday, nontechnical interests of those employing the
concept. The differential explanation account has a clear way
of meeting this point about point: in nondeviant chains the
relevant properties of the experience or action are specifically
explained by the world being as it is or the propositional
attitudes being as they are. When a description of an action or
an experience is explained nondeviantly, the applicability of
those descriptions genuinely mirrors, in a nonreductive way,
the obtaining of truths which employ the distinctive concepts
of the objective world or the agent's propositional attitudes.
The end products of the nondeviant chains give us a glimpse of
these realms as they really are.

5. INTEGRATION

It is an *a posteriori* statement that, for a given scheme of holistic
explanation and field of phenomena to which its application is
in question, there *is* a mechanism with the kind of sensitivity
we have tried to characterize. But the presence of such a
mechanism is epistemically a precondition of applying the
scheme with its distinctive E-concepts at all, in this sense: there
need to be many cases in which conditions producing sensitive
chains actually obtain and produce a bodily movement believed
to be a ϕ-ing (or an experience as of its being ϕ) in order for
us to be able to discern an underlying pattern of beliefs and
desires, or of places and their properties. We already knew, of
course, that it is impossible both for conditions producing
sensitivity to obtain and for a bodily movement believed to be
a ϕ-ing or an experience as of its being ϕ, produced by the
relevant E-truths, not to be respectively intentional or a perception. The present observation is additional both because
(i) it asserts that conditions producing sensitivity must obtain
on many occasions, and (ii) on these occasions the appropriate
B-sentence is caused to be true. (On the 'reliably *matching*'
interpretation of reliability, (ii) was of course not already
ensured: only a conditional was guaranteed.)

This point does not imply that we cannot apply the E-concepts in advance of learning the details of the mechanism: continued success in tentative applications of the E-concepts in respect of truth of predicted B-sentences is itself evidence that there is such a mechanism.[44] If this picture is correct in outline then we may have limited sympathy with the claims of those who have said that in some sense or other there are necessary connections between belief, desire, intention, and action that are not generally present in the physical sciences, while declining to draw the conclusion that the species of explanation employed in the action scheme is noncausal.[45]

What, then, *is* the empirical condition that when substituted for the existentially quantified variable 'C' in the *a priori* condition yields a truth? The observations we made on the possibility of re-routing the causal chains involved in genuine perception or action without destroying the claim of the resulting events to these titles shows clearly that no one condition, not even for a given creature at a given time, formulated in biological and electro-chemical vocabulary, can formulate exhaustively what is necessary and sufficient for nondeviancy of the causal chain. There is no finite number of ways the chain may be modified that exhaust the ways in which the required sensitivity to the belief and desire, or to the state of the place at which the perceiver is located, is preserved. And if we just replaced 'C' with a clause stating that the conditions are fulfilled for genuine perception (perception in modality M) or for intentional action, we seem again to have a resulting principle that is *a priori*. The position here is analogous in some limited respects to the kind of irreducibility we found in the thermostat cases: the condition of being sensitive in the required way, like the general condition of having the function of keeping a certain room at 70°F, is not finitely definable in nonfunctional physical terms (without triviality). But the holding of any one of the infinitely many physical conditions that suffice for the presence of a chain of this kind is expressed

---

[44] It is a matter of scope. It is *a priori* that if a scheme of holistic explanation applies, there are conditions C such that . . . etc. But there are no conditions such that it is *a priori* that if the scheme applied, they are such that . . . etc.

[45] This is not intended to be an account of how the principles can be both *a priori* and have some close relation to principles with an explanatory role: an attempt to deal with this problem will not be made until the next chapter.

in a sentence that can be substituted for 'C' to yield an *a posteriori* conditional. Should we then take *that* conditional as the Hempelian law covering the explanation of action for a given creature at a given time? This question we will defer to the next chapter. The point at present is just that one may have good reasons amounting to knowledge that the scheme applies, without yet kowing of any single detailed physical condition to replace 'C' that is so sufficient: in fact until the sciences of the brain and nervous system are further advanced, that is just our position at present.

I should emphasize strongly that the basis I have suggested for distinguishing deviant from nondeviant chains gives absolutely no nonholistic means of applying the concepts of belief, desire, intention, and so on. The requirement that the agent's intention to ϕ, or its being objectively ϕ, differentially explain a certain effect means that we have already to be able to apply these concepts before we can use the criterion I have suggested. In his essay 'Freedom to Act', Davidson says that he thinks the problem of deviant internal chains 'insurmountable' and that he 'despairs' of spelling out the basis of the distinction.[46] My disagreement with him can be located at the point at which he writes:

to improve on this [naïve causal] formulation, in a way that would eliminate wrong causal chains, would also eliminate the need to depend on the open appeal to causal relations. We would simply say, given these (specified) conditions, there always is an intentional action of a specified type.

My position is that we can appeal to properties of the 'explains' operator rather than the 'causes' relation, and we can do this without appeal to explicit laws of the kind it is clear from his paper Davidson has in mind.

Davidson's worry is that if we did need to appeal to laws saying that under such and such conditions, an intentional action of a certain type would be performed, then either the antecedents of such laws would contain psychological vocabulary, and then they would seem 'constitutive or analytic', or else they would in a broad sense be physical, and then they

---

[46] In *Essays on Freedom of Action* (London: Routledge, 1973), ed. T. Honderich, p. 153.

would violate the position he developed in 'Mental Events'. In the former case, Davidson seems in 'Freedom to Act' to consider only psychological antecedents relating to the agent's desires, rather than his intentions; and the parallel we have developed with perception suggests that there are other examples in which we have on our hands the task of showing how certain principles can be both *a priori* and closely related to explanatory principles.

It should be noted that the principles I have suggested as involved in the explanation of intentional action are not psychophysical laws: the antecedents are partly psychological, but so is the consequent, since it relates to what the agent *takes* to be a ϕ-ing. In the case of perception, matters are more complex, and in this case we do seem to have physical antecedents and a mental consequent about the occurrence of an instance of a certain experience-kind. There are at least three remarks to be made on this. First, though it is easily checked that the 'ϕ' in 'experience as of its being ϕ' is not extensional with respect to predicates occurring in it, to have an experience as of its being ϕ for some particular ϕ is not to have a propositional attitude specified by a 'that' clause: and it appears to be the nonexistence of psychophysical laws about such propositional attitudes that Davidson is most concerned to urge. Second, the conditions that for a given creature are sufficient for his having an experience as of its being ϕ are not also necessary, because of the possibility of re-routing the chains. Third, it is hard to see how there will not be some conditionals giving sufficient physical conditions for an experience as of its being ϕ to occur if, as Davidson himself would hold, mental – and so experience-kind – predicates are supervenient on physical predicates. To say that there is such supervenience is to say that there cannot be two situations agreeing on the application of each physical predicate but differing on the application of some psychological predicate. Now consider the set of all physically possible states of the universe. Each member of this set, that is each physically possible state, will be determinate with respect to what is going of at each spacetime point, which objects are located there and generally the values of physical magnitudes there. If supervenience of the mental on the physical holds, then for any given psychological sentence, the truth value of that sentence will be fixed (not necessarily by translation rules at all) in each one of these possible physical states. At some states the statement that a certain person has a particular kind of experience at a particular time will be true. But if any one of these states at which the statement is true is finitely describable, we can expect there to be a true psychophysical principle stating that in such a state, such an experience occurs. (We take it that differences in the identity of objects unaccompanied by other physical differences does not affect whether the psychological state is exemplified: so much seems to be implied by the definition of supervenience itself.) The psychophysical principle will have a strength determined by the strength of the 'cannot' in the definition of supervenience. It would seem dogmatic to hold that none of the states at which the psychological sentence is true are finitely statable: and though the truth of a psychological predication can depend on the history and environment of the object of which it is predicated, it hardly depends on the whole universe.

Anyone who has followed the argument of this book thus far may naturally be worried by a certain kind of circularity. Let us express the point just for the action case. I said earlier that the E-concepts have to be applied in accordance with the *a priori* principles of their scheme of holistic explanation. Now a causal chain is nondeviant only if it starts with the agent's falling under an E-concept, or something which has to be explained partially in terms of E-concepts. But to check (canonically) that this is so, we have to apply the E-concept in accordance with the *a priori* principle. Does the *a priori* principle contain some feature that in effect restricts the conditions C to nondeviant cases? If it does, then our method of distinguishing deviant from nondeviant chains rests on the presence of some independent criterion of nondeviancy that occurs in the *a priori* principle. If it does not, then the *a priori* principle is incomplete and a notion applied in accordance with it may not coincide with our pretheoretical concept of intention.

The first horn of this alleged dilemma is not correct. It is true that the correct *a priori* principles must contain some means of distinguishing the deviant from the nondeviant chains, but it need not be an 'independent criterion': we may specify the conditions C as those that realize for that person, then, the state of being such that if he intends to ϕ, then he performs a bodily movement of a kind he believes to be a ϕ-ing where this is differentially explained by his intention.

How intimate is the relation between the deviant/nondeviant distinction and the holistic character of a scheme of explanation? Certainly it is not to be denied that if (*per impossibile* if the claims of Chapter I are correct) some nonholistic means could successfully identify beliefs and desires, then a theory incorporating such means could go on at a later stage to take over the account suggested here in terms of differential explanation to distinguish deviant from nondeviant chains. (That is not surprising, since the notion of differential explanation has been defined in terms from the field of explanation generally.) But a more interesting question is whether there is some necessary connection between the features of a scheme of holistic explanation identified as distinctive of the holism in Chapter I and the possibility of introducing a deviant/nondeviant distinction. (I write 'possibility of introducing' here because the fact that a distinction is not in fact marked in the language associated with some explanatory scheme is not of itself for our purposes of any philosophical significance; what is of significance is whether there has to be a distinction that may or may not be marked in the language.) Thus the interesting question is whether a scheme of explanation that is holistic in the sense of Chapter I, section 4, a sense that does not advert explicitly to the availability of a deviant/nondeviant distinction, nevertheless will be one in which such a distinction is introducible. This is to ask whether to add explicitly to the characterization of a holistic scheme of explanation that such a distinction can be drawn is to add an additional requirement not essentially but only accidentally connected with the other characteristics of a scheme of holistic explanation. There are ramifications here beyond the intrinsic interest of the question, because we noted in Chapter I, section 4, that the possibility of drawing such a deviant/nondeviant distinction is something distinguishing the action and spatial schemes from examples of explanation in the physical sciences.

In the next chapter I will suggest an argument for the view that either the E-states or the B-states of a scheme of holistic explanation must be realized by other states, a requirement that seems to be met in the actual world by their realization in the action and spatial cases by states of matter. If some such realization claim has to be true, then a deviant/nondeviant distinction will be essentially connected with the holistic character of the scheme: for we can always introduce a distinction between the cases in which the state that realizes (say) the E-state differentially explains via the physical laws (or analogues thereof) the presence of the relevant B-state, and the cases in which there is no such differential explanation. But if that argument of section 4 of the next chapter is fallacious – and the question is a difficult one, to which none of the obvious answers is entirely satisfactory – then, failing any other argument to the same conclusion, there is no essential connection between the holism of a scheme of explanation and the possibility of drawing a deviant/nondeviant distinction. In that case one would presumably say that the merely contingent fact of physical realization in both the action and spatial cases is sufficient to explain why we in fact draw the deviant/nondeviant distinction in both schemes.

III
PHYSICALISM

1. REALIZATION AND PHYSICALIST THESES

Given the general picture so far presented, what should be said of the relation between the possession of beliefs, desires, and intentions on the one hand and states of the brain on the other? Let us, for the present, allow ourselves to speak in terms that apparently require an ontology of states for their interpretation. Then the consideration, strongly urged in the past by Putnam,[1] that a given psychological state may have many distinct physico-chemical realizations, prevents one from saying that the state of having a certain belief is identical with a state of the brain, where the brain state is canonically specified in physico-chemical vocabulary. Nevertheless if the above account of holistic explanation is correct and action explanation is a case of it, there is an obvious argument to show that there must be an intimate relation between the two states. We will assume for the present that beliefs and desires or intentions do explain token actions under some or other of their descriptions; a defence of this supposition, which is by no means unquestionable, will be offered later in this chapter. If the supposition is true, then the particular token actions explained under some description by the possession of beliefs and desires are, in the strict sense of identity, physical events, bodily movements in the general case. Where ϕ is the description under which an action is thus intentionally explained, on a particular occasion only certain of the movements physically open to an agent (in virtue of his strength, size, and so forth) will be ϕ-ings; hence the

[1] See, for instance, 'The Mental Life of Some Machines' and 'The Nature of Mental States', both reprinted in Putnam's *Mind, Language and Reality*, Philosophical Papers, vol. ii (Cambridge: CUP, 1975). By 'states' I should make clear that I mean type and not 'token' states: obviously Putnam's considerations do not tell against token state identity theses. I suspect that talk about token states can be translated into talk about the realization relation I discuss below; in particular it is plausible that the token state of x's being ϕ is identical with the token state of y's being ψ iff x's being ϕ is realized by y's being ψ. Further, if there are counterexamples to the notion of realization below, given the theoretical role it is intended to play, I would expect these counterexamples also to make plausible a different identity condition for token states – if indeed one has to be given at all.

physical antecedents of the actual ϕ-ing on that occasion must at least be sufficient to give rise to consequences that are ϕ-ings. But the crucial components of the physical antecedents of the actual ϕ-ing is the state of the brain; so the explanatory presence of a belief and a desire must in the circumstances at least involve the brain being in one of a circumscribed set of states; and the restrictions must be more severe when we take into account the fact that any given desire may combine with any one of a potentially infinite set of beliefs in producing action.

One relation between attitudes and states of the brain which is weaker than type–type identity, but which might provide the right sort of close connection, is the relation of realization. The basic notion here, expressed just for the purely monadic case, is 'x's being ϕ is realized by y's being ψ'. What I have to say about realization will easily generalize to predications of greater degree; and the label should be drained of any associations it may have with functionalist doctrines in the philosophy of mind. (The notion of realization with which I am concerned will be available equally to functionalists and to those who are not functionalists.) Let us have some examples of this concept before giving a definition:

(i) a and b's being in direct contact is realized by there being an open line between their telephones:

(ii) a pocket calculator's having a multiplication facility is realized by its having a printed circuit of a certain kind;

(iii) my bank's having a record that I have £100 with them is realized by a certain pattern being recorded on a section of magnetic tape in their computer.

In none of these examples (i)–(iii) does the fact that x's being ϕ is realized by y's being ψ justify the claim that necessarily any object that is ϕ is ψ.

There is, though, a more restricted class of contexts with respect to which the concept of realization sustains substitution, and these are causal contexts. If x's being ϕ is realized by y's being ψ, then the facts that $\phi(x)$ and that $\psi(y)$ have their causes and effects in common. Indeed, we shall *define* the notion of realization as the indiscernibility relation with respect to causal contexts of a sentential kind. Let 'CTB' abbreviate 'causes it to be the case that', an operator taking a pair of sentences, indifferently closed or open, to yield a sentence that will be open if one of the sentences upon which it operates is open. Then the intuitive idea is to say, where '$\forall\chi$' is a primitive substitutional quantifier over sentences,

x's being ϕ is realized by y's being ψ iff:

$$\forall\chi(\chi CTB\phi(x) \equiv \chi CTB\psi(y)) \ \& \ \forall\chi(\phi(x)CTB\chi \equiv \psi(y)CTB\chi)$$

(This is simply an adaptation to the sentential case of a criterion of identity for events suggested by Thomas Nagel.[2]) The definition I have just given is in need of some technical refinements, but I will relegate these to a footnote.[3]

Thus, in our example (i), if a telephone operator's pressing a button caused there to be an open telephone line between a and b, he caused them to be in direct contact. Similarly, under the realization suggestion, any causes or effects of a human being's having a belief, desire, or intention will be causes or effects of his brain's being in a certain state. If that is so, it would allow the truth of such slightly odd sentences as 'John's belief that the year is 1977 caused the concentration of substance A to rise in area R of his brain.' But the oddity here may be occasioned by the unusual (and of course explanatorily useless) combination of levels of description; and this is no more a bar to its literal truth than it is in the case of 'John's

[2] 'Physicalism', *Philosophical Review* 74 (1965): 346-7. Note that I have not defined realization in terms of satisfaction of a theory, in the way David Lewis does in 'Psychophysical and Theoretical Identifications', *Australasian Journal of Philosophy* 50 (1972): 249-58; it is a substantial claim that the two definitions have the same extension in the psychological case.

[3] The definition is inadequate for two reasons. The more serious difficulty is that there is an undesirable relativity to the expressive power of our language: if two states of an object at a given time had exactly the same causes and effects as expressed by the CTB operator using the vocabulary of our present language, then by such a definition one would be counted as realizing the other (for the given object at the given time), even if it were the case that in a language with a richer stock of predicates, something could be identified as the cause of the object's being in one state but not the other (and similarly for effects). A second difficulty with the definition is that we obviously need to permit as substituends for 'χ' sentences with expressions functioning as free variables.

We can meet both these difficulties simultaneously as follows. Let an extension of English be any language just like English except possibly in containing additional proper names for objects not already named in English and additional predicates for properties not expressed in English. Then to say that x's being ϕ is realized by y's being ψ is to say that for any language L that is an extension of English and for any closed sentnece χ of L, $\langle x,y \rangle$ satisfies in L the expression

$\ulcorner(\chi CTB\phi(\zeta_1) \equiv \chi CTB\psi(\zeta_2)) \ \& \ (\phi(\zeta_1)CTB\chi \equiv \psi(\zeta_2)CTB\chi)\urcorner$.

seeing a red flash caused the cone cells of his retina to contain chemical C two seconds later (as an after-effect).'

The causal contexts with respect to which such a realization relation sustains substitution will include, for instance, '—— caused it to be the case that John raised his arm'. This answers a point raised in an extraordinary paper by Norman Malcolm entitled 'The Conceivability of Mechanism', in which he maintains that if a complete neurophysiological explanation could be given of a particular action, a man's intentions, beliefs, and desires would then be irrelevant to its explanation.[4] The only ways, he says, in which one could deny this would be to be a state–state identity theorist, an epiphenomenalist, or a logical behaviourist.[5] Understandably finding these unattractive, he takes the short step to the conclusion that mechanism is inconceivable as things actually are.[6] But of course Malcolm's disjunction is not exhaustive: a neural state N and a propositional attitude P may be related in such a way, in particular by the realization relation, that if John's having P caused it to be the case that John raised his arm, then John's being in N caused it to be the case that John raised his arm; and so we cannot argue from the fact that the presence of state N is necessary and sufficient for the agent to have acted as he did to the conclusion that his psychological state is irrelevant to accounting for his action. We can make this point without being state–state identity theorists, epiphenomenalists, or logical behaviourists. In terms of our earlier example, we do not need to take up the analogues of any of those positions in order to maintain that it is a *non sequitur* to move from 'The existence of an open telephone line between a and b helped the speedy formation of an agreement between them' to 'The fact that a and b were in direct contact was irrelevant to the speed with which agreement was reached.'[7]

[4] *Philosophical Review* 77 (1968): 45-72.

[5] Ibid., pp. 53-5.

[6] But see his sudden doubts, no doubt because of the strength of his conclusion, ibid., p. 72.

[7] The fact that a realization relation between states can be defined without any commitment to the reducibility of psychological predicates to others, means that I am bound to disagree with the import of such statements as this by Dennett (*Content and Consciousness* [London: Routledge, 1969], pp. 35-6):

'It follows directly from the Intentionalist's irreducibility hypothesis that no independent characterization of an Intentionally characterized antecedent is

The particular examples (i)–(iii) have a property in common besides the one already noted. In each case, the condition that is said to be the realizing condition describes a unique object which verifies an existential quantification in the condition presented as realized by it. Thus the pattern on the magnetic tape may be said to *be* the record which the realized condition in (iii) says that the bank has. This has the consequence that if such realization claims as (i)–(iii) are true, it has to be the case that if there is something, b say, that is uniquely F, then for any p, $(\exists! x\, Fx$ causes it to be the case that p) iff (Fb causes it to be the case that p). That principle seems to be acceptable: if for example there is just one drop of water (b, say) in the machine, the fact that there is a drop of water in the machine causes a short circuit if and only if the presence of that particular drop b causes the short circuit. One natural speculation is that all nontrivial cases of realization have this structure of existential quantification and particular instance. I shall not discuss this further here, except to note that in the case of propositional attitudes it would be natural to link this suggestion to the idea that in certain circumstances we can make sense of the possibility that one man has two beliefs that (say) there are snakes in England. Consider a man who (let us suppose) both is a zoologist and takes his family camping in England, and who has acquired the belief that there are snakes in England in two different connections: if there is some compartmentalization of his beliefs, so that on each occasion of acquisition the acquisition has inferential consequences only for beliefs in the compartment associated with that occasion of acquisition, it is possible to think of empirical evidence that one and not the other belief has disappeared, or is explaining his current actions, and so forth.

Suppose we take the claim that all objects are physical to be the conjunction of the claims that every physical object consists wholly of entities of which the predicates of fundamental

---

ever possible. To say that a particular Intentionally characterized antecedent could be characterized in another way is to say that either the Intentional sentence announcing the occurrence of this antecedent has an extensional paraphrase (and this is ruled out *ex hypothesi*), or the Intentionally characterized antecedent can be given a different Intentional characterization, but this is contrary to the fundamental principle of Intentionality . . .'

physics are true, and that every token event is a sum of the events quantified over in fundamental physics. Now if we hold that all objects are physical objects in that sense, and that every psychological state is realized by some physico-chemical state, and that every relation not definable in physico-chemical and logical vocabulary is at least supervenient on physico-chemical relations, is that the strongest form of physicalism with respect to psychological predicates in which we have any right to believe? Or is something stronger true? And if so, is what is extra, something that can hold only if some form of reductionism is true, or is there a weaker extra condition? The extra will not of course in a strict sense be a doctrine of ontology. It would also not be correct to say that such a form of physicalism is silent about the concept of explanation: for the doctrine about realization makes commitments about explanation. Nevertheless I shall briefly argue that there is another element in a plausible physicalism that is omitted from the description just given.

A first point to note which encourages the thought that something has been omitted is the observation that if the realization relation is simply defined as the (or an) indiscernibility relation with respect to certain causal contexts, with nothing more required, then there is nothing intrinsically asymmetrical about that relation: on such a definition, for a given sequence of objects at a given time, its psychological states will be realized by certain of its physical states, but it will equally be true that those physical states are realized by the psychological states, if indiscernibility is all that is required in the definition. For instance, to see how weak this doctrine of realization is, we may note that all of the ontological realization and supervenience doctrines may be simultaneously true, yet it also be the case that psychological generalizations are explanatorily fundamental in the sense that it is their truth alone which circumscribes from initial conditions the later positions of the fundamental particles of matter. This would still be compatible with supervenience of psychological upon physical statements, for that does not require any explanatory primacy of the class of statements upon which others are said to be supervenient: no such primacy is implied by the claim that there cannot be two situations alike in all physical respects but differing in some psychological respect.

Here a parallel may be helpful. Someone may hold that there are laws governing the behaviour of nations. He may hold that these laws, which may for instance predict that there will be a war between a certain pair of nations in the next few years, in no way require a particular determinate pattern of behaviour of each citizen of the nations in those years: the law merely rules out all total patterns that do not yield the result that the nations are at war. It seems clear that such a man could consistently hold along with this view both that all statements about nations are supervenient upon psychological and semantic statements about individual citizens of nations, and that every event in which a nation participates is an event consisting wholly of events in which only individual citizens participate, and that every state in which a nation might be is realized, for given objects at a given time, by a state canonically specified by propositional attitude vocabulary. (I write of the consistency of such a position, not its plausibility.) It seems to me that we are in a position to propose a version of physicalism stronger than one which is just a psychological analogue of this man's views on statements about nations.[8]

---

[8] Would this kind of example be ruled out by the requirement that truths about individual citizens (physics) *determine* truths about nations (psychology) in the sense of G. Hellman and F. Thompson ('Physicalism: Ontology, Determination, and Reduction', *Journal of Philosophy* 72 (1975): 558)? Their definition is:
  In a structures, ϕ truth determines ψ truth
  iff
  for any models m and m' both in the set a of structures, if m restricted to ϕ vocabulary is elementarily equivalent to m' restricted to ϕ vocabulary then m and m' both restricted to ψ vocabulary are elementarily equivalent.
(Here ϕ and ψ are sets of nonlogical expressions.) The set of structures a intuitively represents genuine possibilities – at very least, we would require its members to be models of accepted scientific theory. It is also important that, in the theory we require all members of a to model, all *supervenience conditionals* should be included: that is, all true lawlike universally quantified conditionals with physical antecedents and mental consequents. Even with these conditions met, however, it seems that the requirement of determination would not exclude the kind of example given in the text: for this determination requirement in no way involves that the physical laws have properties that are not symmetrically possessed by psychological laws, and this was what produced the asymmetry we wished to capture. Indeed it seems that supervenience is sufficient for Hellman–Thompson determination, and since in our nation example and its psychological analogue, supervenience holds but the property we wish to capture is not present, determination cannot help us.
  It may be noted that the set of all supervenience conditionals may well not be recursively enumerable, and so Hellman and Thompson's worry (ibid., p. 562)

There is a further principle that it is plausible to assert as a high-level empirical hypothesis, confirmed by the findings of many sciences, and I shall call it the Principle of Physical Embedding. Roughly, it asserts that if ψ_1 and ψ_2 are each psychological descriptions of objects or events x and y respectively, and it is true that x's being ψ_1 causes y's being ψ_2, then there are descriptions ϕ_1 and ϕ_2 each composed of only physical and logical vocabulary such that it is a consequence of physical theory, given some other physical initial conditions, that x's being ϕ_1 explains y's being ϕ_2. (The laws used in this physical theory are *a posteriori*, or, if they are like the cases considered earlier in Chapter I in which the laws are *a priori*, there is no possibility of a distinction between deviant and nondeviant causal chains in the application of these *a priori* principles.) Note that it is not required that x's being ϕ_1 is *sufficient* according to the physical theory in the circumstances for y's being ϕ_2: there is certainly some notion of explanation according to which we can explain why a plutonium atom fired out the particles it does, and in particular be entitled to say that if the atom had not been present, the particles would not, without implying that in any similar circumstances similar particles would have been fired out. (This is a now familiar point in recent accounts of causation.) There is also a point omitted in the above statement of the Principle of Physical Embedding: we also require that in the circumstances, the descriptions ψ_1 and ψ_2 be supervenient on the descriptions ϕ_1 and ϕ_2 respectively.[9] It should in any case be clear that with or without that addition, physical and psychological predicates are asymmetrically related in the Principle of Physical Embedding. Note that our imagine theorist of the explanation of the behaviour of nations would not hold true an analogous principle of embedding relating descriptions of the actions of nations to descriptions of the propositional attitudes of citizens

---

that Determination will collapse into Reducibility (via Beth's Definability Theorem) if the set α is the set of all and only the models of a first-order theory, could be answered without appeal to nonstandard models.

[9] In this sentence, 'in the circumstances' is present because we wish to allow that the description ψ_1 may not supervene on ϕ_1 until various physical truths about the surrounding environment are given. We would of course require these extra truths not to be such that ψ_1 would supervene upon them regardless of whether ϕ_1 applied.

as psychological and physical descriptions are related by the Principle of Physical Embedding.

The Principle of Physical Embedding is also entirely non-reductive; it carries no implication that there are reducing formulae that preserve nomologicality and carry one in general from psychological to nonpsychological predicates. 'In general' here means: for every occasion, for any physically possible creature to whom we would ascribe propositional attitudes.

2. KRIPKE'S OBJECTIONS

I will continue this chapter by considering Kripke's objections to physicalism.[10] Kripke's objections apply to any phenomenological notion. From what I have already said it follows that belief, desire, and intention are not purely phenomenological notions: so what is the relevance of Kripke's objections? First, anyone who thinks there are at least phenomenological components in the E-concepts of the action scheme and who also finds Kripke's objections compelling will be dissatisfied with the mild physicalism of the previous section. Second, if Kripke's objections are correct, we cannot accept accounts of the relation between the physical and the psychological that are based on the idea that there are token physical events or states that fall under psychologically irreducible descriptions. If Kripke's objections are correct, some quite different prototype must be used: and may this new prototype not apply equally to belief, desire, and intention? But quite apart from these motivations Kripke's objections are of the greatest intrinsic interest.

I ought to make it clear that Kripke said that he had by no means considered all possible replies to his arguments, and that some at least of the arguments for some kinds of identity theory he found difficult to answer. So some parts of what I have to say may not even be in conflict with what Kripke actually believed in 1970, let alone what he holds today.

Kripke's objections are sufficiently well known not to need detailed exposition. The heart of his case against identity theories is that the explanation that can be given of the illusion of contingency of what is in fact a necessary (but *a posteriori*) truth that heat is molecular motion will not carry over to show

[10] 'Naming and Necessity' in *Semantics of Natural Language*, eds. D. Davidson and G. Harman (Dordrecht: Reidel, 1972).

that the apparent contingency of the truths of an identity theory is also illusory. If we feel an inclination to count it as contingent that heat is molecular motion, this inclination is to be explained, Kripke says, by the contingency that what produces in us a certain sensation is in fact the motion of molecules. Molecular motion might be present without the presence of the sensation that is actually the sensation of heat; conversely, something other than molecular motion (heat) might have produced the sensation that is the sensation we actually obtain from heat, so that equally the sensation could be present without molecular motion being present. It is worth making this explanation of the illusion of contingency very explicit. In this section we will use '⟨E⟩' for 'it is epistemically possible that' or 'it could apparently turn out that', and '⟨R⟩' for real ('metaphysical') possibility. Then the illusion is being explained thus: the truth of

$$\langle E \rangle \sim (\text{heat} = \text{molecular motion})$$

is explained by the truth of

$$\langle R \rangle \text{ (molecular motion is present and the sensation of heat is not present)}.$$

Kripke's argument, at least in the type–type case, is that a similar attempt to explain away the appearance of contingency of the identity theory is impossible.[11] For if we say that

$$\langle E \rangle \sim (\text{C-fibre stimulation} = \text{pain})$$

and then proceed as in the case of heat to say that this is true because

$$\langle R \rangle \text{ (C-fibre stimulation is present and the sensation of pain is not present)}$$

then we have reached a formula that is actually incompatible with the identity theory: the reason is that if the identity theory is true, then for the sensation of pain to be present is for pain to be present, and conversely. So that last displayed condition actually implies that

$$\langle R \rangle \text{ (C-fibre stimulation is present and pain is not present)}$$

[11] 'Naming and Necessity', p. 339.

– something no identity theorist of the kind in question could accept if he is clear-headed about identity and necessity. So on Kripke's views the identity theorist cannot admit even the epistemic possibility that C-fibre stimulation is not pain. The difference between the heat and the pain cases is that while the sensation of heat can be present independently of the physical phenomenon that heat is, this is not true of pain, which is apparently a purely phenomenological notion. (It is true that we sometimes speak in ways that might appear to commit us to the possibility of the existence of pain without the sensation of pain – 'I was so interested in what he was saying that I did not notice my continuing pain' – but whatever the status of such sentences, there can be no objection to Kripke's introducing a more purely phenomenological concept of pain than the English word 'pain' in fact expresses. For the newly introduced notion, Kripke's argument still stands, and it was for such a purely phenomenological notion that the identity theory was of real interest.)

The claim that the materialist is committed to the real and not merely the epistemic possibility that C-fibre stimulation can exist without the sensation of pain existing is no mere optional extra that could be dropped from Kripke's main argument without any loss of force. It is an essential component of his case that the identity theorist cannot explain away the illusion of contingency in the way that is possible for the man who maintains that it is necessary that heat is molecular motion. If it could be shown that it is too strong in general to require a real rather than an epistemic possibility in explaining illusions of contingency, then the argument, that the materialist in question cannot accept even the epistemic possibility that C-fibre stimulation can exist without the presence of the sensation of pain, will not go through. (Perhaps, of course, the argument can be reformulated; we will look at a few suggestions later.) But *prima facie* if the requirement is too strong, then the identity theory might be one of the cases in which a corresponding real possibility is not entailed by the epistemic possibility.

My strategy in suggesting a reply to Kripke's objections will be to distinguish two putative explanations of the illusions of contingency. Though these explanations agree in some cases on the explanation of the illusion, they disagree in others, and so are rivals for our assent. I shall call the two explanations 'the reference fixing explanation' and 'the qualitative explanation', and I will argue that the first is incorrect, while the second is not incompatible with the identity theory if consistently applied.

Suppose we have a true, metaphysically necessary identity $\alpha = \beta$, and we have also the illusion of contingency:

$\quad$ Ⓔ $\quad \sim (\alpha = \beta)$.

Suppose the name α has as reference fixing description 'the ϕ', and that β has as its reference fixing description 'the ψ'. Then the fundamental claim of the reference fixing explanation is that the illusion of contingency of the identity $\alpha = \beta$ has its source in the truth that

$\quad$ Ⓡ $\quad \sim (\text{the } \phi = \text{the } \psi)$.

(Here the two definite descriptions have narrower scope than 'Ⓡ' but wider scope than '$\sim$'.) There are several possible variants of the reference fixing explanation: for example, if we are concerned with epistemic possibility for a particular person at a particular time, then one variant of the reference fixing explanation will make us look to some favoured descriptions the person will offer in answer to the questions 'What is α?' and 'What is β?'

The qualitative explanation on the other hand claims that the explanation of the illusion of contingency is that, where $Q(\phi)$ and $Q(\psi)$ in some way express corresponding qualitative predicates related to ϕ and ψ, it is true that

$\quad$ Ⓡ $\quad \sim (\text{the } Q(\phi) = \text{the } Q(\psi))$

Again, the descriptions have intermediate scope. It is not easy to explain generally what is meant by 'corresponding qualitative predicate' here. Certainly a qualitative predicate (simple or complex) must not contain natural kind words not embedded in 'seems', 'looks', or 'feels', nor may they contain proper names of individuals. I will take it that the reader has a firm enough grasp on the notion of a qualitative predicate from the writings of Kripke for discussion to proceed.

Clearly the reference fixing explanation and the qualitative explanation will coincide if the reference fixing descriptions of the names α and β use only qualitative predicates, but otherwise they will diverge. A case in which they in effect coincide (since any nonqualitative elements in the sense of the predicates are the same in both cases) is in the explanation of the illusion of contingency of 'Hesperus = Phosphorus': both explanations agree that the source of the illusion is that

⑧ ~(the heavenly body to appear last in the morning = the heavenly body to appear first in the evening).

But in other cases the explanations diverge.

Consider a scientist who introduces two substance names γ and δ. He fixes their references thus: γ is to denote the substance that, together with salt, is produced by the reaction of hydrochloric acid and sodium hydroxide in equal parts ($HCl + NaOH \rightarrow NaCl + H_2O$); while δ is to denote the substance occurring naturally in liquid form on earth that is needed by plants and human beings to live. This scientist, we are to suppose, does not know whether the same substance satisfies these two descriptions; so given these circumstances we have to say that (perhaps relative to that scientist, then)

⟨E⟩ ~$(\gamma = \delta)$.

According to the reference fixing explanation, this is because it is true that

⟨E⟩ $\exists S\, \exists S'$ (S is the substance needed by humans to live and S' is the substance that results in the specified reaction and ~$S = S'$).

Now is this a real possibility? On the grounds supplied by the theory of natural kinds of Kripke and Putnam, human beings necessarily have the internal constitution they do, and the liquid *they* need to live could not be other than water; nor can the liquid produced in the given chemical reaction be other than water, where this 'can' is the 'can' of metaphysical possibility. Hence there is no really possible circumstance in which some substance is both needed by humans and is not produced in that reaction. Since in this example an epistemic possibility claim is true but the corresponding real possibility statement given by the reference fixing explanation is false, that explanation appears to be incorrect. (Those who doubt that human beings necessarily need water to live may change the example to one in which δ denotes the substance (water, in fact) which results from some other chemical reaction.)

One conclusion one might draw from this example is that the corresponding statement does not have to be really possible but only epistemically possible. (A conclusive argument for replacing '⟨R⟩' by '⟨E⟩' in the qualitative explanation would be given by an example in which what are apparently two properties have different associated qualitative descriptions, and where these two qualitative descriptions are equivalent as a matter of *a posteriori* necessity.) Obviously the suggestion offers no prospect of a general reduction of epistemic possibility to something else, but only a connection between two of its applications.)[12]

The defender of the qualitative explanation will not be surprised at this outcome, and will say that the defender of the reference fixing explanation has simply been appealing to the wrong possibility statement. The reference fixing descriptions for γ and δ in the example we have given contain such natural kind words as 'NaCl': this, for instance, should be replaced by 'white crystalline substance with a salty taste'. When we carry through this policy, the qualitative explanation offers us as the explanation of the illusion of contingency the claim that

⟨R⟩ $\exists S \, \exists S'$ (S is the substance needed by anthropoid-looking creatures to live and S' is the substance with a salty taste, etc., and $\sim S = S'$).

This is indeed true, as the qualitative explanation requires; and its truth is also intuitively the source of the illusion of contingency.

This offers some confirmation of the qualitative explanation. How does the qualitative explanation fare with 'C-fibre

---

[12] It may be asked why I have not simply used the example of arithmetical computations whose outcome is not known in advance in order to show that the qualitative contingency claim is not generally true. The reason is that in these examples it may be said that epistemic possibility of p just involves it not being known that not-p: and this is of course compatible with one's knowing that when one carries out an investigation, all the principles and rules of inference one uses either have or preserve the property of necessary truth. But in empirical cases this is not so: indeed the principle that $x = y \supset \Box(x = y)$ is *a priori* and itself necessary, but it is not the necessitation of some principle one uses in establishing that (for instance) Hesperus is Phosphorus, nor are all the other truths discovered in an investigation leading to the discovery of that identity *a priori* and necessary. Thus there would be a natural restriction of the qualitative contingency claim that would make it immune in the restricted form to arithmetical counterexamples of that kind.

stimulation = pain'? We must replace 'C-fibre' with some description such as 'strand of grey fibrous cells of such and such shape', and then consider the statement

    Ⓡ (strands of grey fibrous cells of such and such shape are stimulated and pain is absent).

But this is *true*, since presumably strands of grey . . . etc. are not necessarily C-fibres. So the qualitative explanation does not go against the identity theorist who makes a claim of an *a posteriori* identity of C-fibres with pain. Note also that he can say that truth is preserved when 'C-fibre stimulation' is substituted for 'pain' in the last displayed statement.

It might be replied on behalf of Kripke that in, for instance, 'Hesperus is Phosphorus', it is sufficient to replace *one* of the names in the identity by a qualitative description to obtain a genuinely contingent truth. If this were the explanation, it then need not carry over to explain an illusion of contingency in the case of 'C-fibre stimulation = pain', since 'pain' is already qualitative, and no replacement is needed. However this reply will not work. Consider 'Heat = molecular motion'. As Kripke is well aware, it might turn out to be *a posteriori* necessary that molecular motion produces in us the sensation of heat. Hence the explanation of the illusion must be the genuine contingency of the qualitative statement when *both* terms are replaced, as in, for instance, 'Whatever looks such and such way under such and such kind of instrument (qualitatively specified) causes in us the sensation of heat.'

The qualitative theory certainly needs more elaboration. In particular, something must be said about demonstratives, for there is certainly an illusion of contingency in some utterances containing demonstratives on each side of the identity sign. Perhaps in some of these cases the theory should make use of the notion of the sense of a demonstration in the sense introduced by Kaplan.[13] There may be yet other cases in which it is impossible to find an appropriate qualitative statement corresponding to the illusion of contingency. But the explanation offered by the qualitative theory when there are such statements has great plausibility: this would not preclude the explanation

[13] At the time of writing, Kaplan's theory is still unpublished. I follow the text of 'Demonstratives' prepared for the Pacific Division meetings of the APA in 1977.

from being an instance of some more generally applicable formula.

There are other, weaker, theories that might be offered to explain the illusion of contingency. Another example of a theory that either is too strong or else is consistent with the identity theory is one that emphasizes that the fundamental notion is that of its being epistemically possible for person x at time t that A. Nothing, it may be said, in the examples I have given is incompatible with the view that it is epistemically possible for x at t that A iff x believes that the corresponding statement containing descriptions cited by the reference fixing theory is metaphysically possible. But that condition would be too strong for epistemic possibility: if, for instance, our scientist accepted Kripke's theory of metaphysical possibility, then even though for him in advance of investigation it is epistemically possible that γ is not δ, he will not be prepared to believe that it is metaphysically possible that γ is not δ until the outcome of his empirical investigation is clear. Perhaps then the appropriate definition is this: it is not the case that x believes at t that the qualitative analogue of A is *not* metaphysically possible. The case we looked at two sentences back would not be a counterexample to *that* definition. But does this definition (or indeed the one just rejected) give much leverage against the identity theorist? Certainly a type–type identity theorist who is not confused will now believe that it is not metaphysically possible for C-fibres to be stimulated and the sensation of pain not to be present. But he may still fairly say that for all he knew in the past, it might have turned out that pain is not stimulation of C-fibres: he may say this because the past tense makes the epistemic possibility relative to his earlier body of information, prior to his acceptance of any argument for the identity theory. He may say this, much as someone who accepts both Kripke's account of metaphysical possibility and that Hesperus is Phosphorus may say that for all he knew earlier, it might have turned out that Hesperus is not Phosphorus.[14]

---

[14] In his 1974 paper ('What is it Like to be a Bat?', *Philosophical Review* 81 (1974): 445–6) Nagel offers a different criticism of Kripke's argument, a criticism founded on the idea that two kinds of imagination, which Nagel calls 'perceptual' and 'sympathetic', are independent of one another. How are his criticism and mine related? Where 'Px' abbreviates 'x is in pain' and 'Bx' abbreviates 'x is in brain state B', let us consider the assessment of the truth value of the sentence:

In order to avoid misunderstanding of the position I wish to defend, I will make some comments on the arguments presented so far. The first comment is that it may truly be said that none of the examples I have presented, in which the move from epistemic possibility to real possibility of a corresponding statement fails, is a case in which the reference of the relevant term is fixed by the fact that a certain property or magnitude is one which uniquely produces a certain sensation in us, or indeed *is* a term for a conscious mental state. Yet 'pain' is conspicuously such a case. So may not the qualitative contingency claim be restricted to just such cases, and thus be made immune to the examples we have given? My view is that the implication from epistemic to corresponding real possibility cannot be assessed outside the context of a total theory of the relations between mental and physical events and states. I shall soon offer an argument which I will claim can carry us from empirical premises that we may have reason to believe true to the conclusion that a kind of token–token identity theory is true. If those empirical premises are indeed true, we may well come to the conclusion that in order to make all our beliefs consistent with one another our best course is to hold that the implication from epistemic possibility to a certain corresponding real possibility fails even when the terms in question are terms for conscious mental states.[15]

---

it is epistemically possible that (*Px* and $\sim Bx$).

Where this is assessed by perceptual imagination of '*B*' and sympathetic imagination of '*P*', Nagel will deny that the epistemic possibility of the embedded sentence implies its genuine ('real') possibility; so it is not in general the case, according to Nagel, that a sentence of the form 'it is epistemically possible that *p*' implies the corresponding sentence of the form 'it is really possible that *p*'. So far the comments of Nagel and my own are in step. But the example in the text of water and the liquid produced in a certain reaction, in which in the epistemic possibility in question the imagination would in both cases be perceptual, suggests that independence of the two kinds is not by itself the explanation of the failure of epistemic possibility to imply real possibility. If (as of course there may not be) there is a uniform explanation of the failure of this implication, it must be something more general than the independence of perceptual and sympathetic imagination; this is not of course to say that the difference between these two kinds is not a special case of the more general explanation.

[15] I would similarly say that if the empirical premises are established which, it is argued below, entail a token–token identity theory, then the total theory may make it reasonable to say that either a token pain event is not essentially a pain, or that (less unreasonably) a token brain event *is* essentially a pain.

The second comment is that though I have criticized an argument that purported to refute a type–type identity theory, I hold no brief for such theories. It is just that the (familiar) objections to them lie elsewhere.[16]

Third, Kripke might insist that it is *true* that it is really possible for C-fibre stimulation to exist and pain to be absent. All I have been concerned to show in this section is that if it is a real possibility, it is not one that follows from the epistemic possibility that C-fibre stimulation is not pain by itself. Against someone who insists that it *is* a real possibility, we need some argument that will force us to reinterpret such an intuition of real possibility just as we are possessed of arguments that force us to reinterpret an intuition that Hesperus might not have been Phosphorus. Such an argument will be suggested in the next section, for the token–token case.

I will now turn to suggest an argument with empirical premises that we could have reason for believing and that would imply the truth of a psychophysical identity theory. Kripke remarks at one point that 'a philosopher who wishes to refute the Cartesian conclusion must refute the Cartesian premise, and the latter task is not trivial.'[17] Now the reason that we hold that in no possible world are Hesperus and Phosphorus distinct is because we have empirically established an identity. Analogously we may hope to block the Cartesian argument not by attacking the first premise of a Cartesian

---

[16] It may alternatively be asked why I have not simply followed the argument of Colin McGinn's note, 'Anomalous Monism and Kripke's Cartesian Intuitions', *Analysis* 37 (1976–7): 78–80. The reason is that one can imagine a Kripkean insisting that his intuition concerning a token brain event is that that very token event might not have been a pain event, and not just that some epistemic counterpart of it is not; the case is different from that of the lectern, he may say, because in that case we have an idea, given the thesis of the necessity of origin, of how further empirical information can show of a particular lectern that it could not (say) have had a different origin, or have been made originally of something different. Hence we are obliged to reinterpret the intuitive claim that that lectern could have turned out to have had a different origin. But nothing, such a theorist may continue, obliges us to reinterpret the modal intuition about the brain event: we have no idea, he may say, of how further empirical information would show that that event could not but be a pain event. The next section of the text is intended to show how empirical information may entail just that. In one sense, then, what follows tends to support McGinn's position, because it shows that the modal intuition cannot be taken at face value; and uniformity with the lectern case will incline us to interpret it in some counterpart fashion, as he suggests.

[17] 'Naming and Necessity', p. 335.

argument directly, but by finding empirical premises from which the identity follows, and then proceeding to argue contrapositively to the falsity of the Cartesian conclusion.

3. AN ARGUMENT FOR TOKEN IDENTITY

Suppose you touch a hot kettle and the pain causes you to withdraw your hand. Let this token pain event be c_ψ, and let the token event that is the effect, the withdrawal of the hand, be e; and suppose that there is a certain event c_ϕ that occurs in your nervous system at the same time as the pain event and that is a cause of the bodily movement e of withdrawal.[18] About c_ϕ we will make two empirical suppositions. The first is that we have a complete and wholly physical account of both the causal antecedents of c_ϕ and also of the causal route from c_ϕ to e in neurophysiological terms; this account completely explains how the event c_ϕ causes e. The second supposition is that the event c_ϕ is the only physical event occurring at the time it actually does that causes the bodily movement e (we are not excluding as causes nonphysical events occurring at that time). These are strong assumptions that we could know only by detailed empirical investigation; but it is hard to believe that a scientist *could* not come to know them. I claim that we have enough resources, when combined with commonplaces about the interaction of the mental and physical in examples like this one, to demonstrate that $c_\phi = c_\psi$.[19]

---

[18] In fact in many such cases the bodily movement of withdrawal is a reflex, and both it and the only event in the brain that might plausibly be identical with c_ψ are caused by an event in the spinal cord. We must consider a case in which the reflex mechanism is not operative. Even if the reflex mechanism were *always* operative, we could apply the argument to a different physical event that is a consequence of c_φ, say a wince on the face. Any token event will serve the function of e in this example provided only that (a) it is a physical event, (b) it is caused by the pain event c_ψ, and (c) it would not have occurred if c_φ had not occurred.

[19] In 'The Uniqueness in Causation' (*American Philosophical Quarterly* 14 (1977): 177–88), Peter Unger has made a plausible case for the principle that any cause of a particular effect must be unique. He would say that in the case of over-determination of an effect e by events c_1 and c_2, the Goodmanian sum of c_1 and c_2 causes e: the difference between overdetermination and joint sufficiency is that in the former if either c_1 or c_2 had not occurred, the other would have caused e, and this is not true in a case of joint sufficiency. If Unger's claim is accepted, 'causes' in the text should be read as 'is a part of the cause of', the way in fact that Unger reads 'is *a* cause of'. (I am not endorsing Unger's views on the relevance of ellipsis to the interpretation of sentences like 'John caused Jim's death'.)

Let us assume for *reductio* that c_ϕ is not identical with c_ψ. Then only two cases can arise: either (1) c_ϕ and c_ψ are jointly sufficient for e but do not overdetermine it, or else (2) e is overdetermined by c_ϕ and c_ψ.

Case (1) is impossible under our assumptions: for they included the supposition that we had a complete physical account of the causal route from c_ϕ to e, an account that did not need to include any nonphysical causes. If there were only joint sufficiency of c_ϕ and c_ψ for e, then it would be true that if c_ψ had not occurred, then e would not have occurred, and so no such complete physical account would be available. (I will consider some objections to this below.)

Case (2), that of overdetermination, is also impossible. Overdetermination implies that even if the pain event had not occurred, the withdrawal of the hand would still have occurred (again, we ignore fail-safe mechanisms). This we certainly ordinarily take to be false,[20] and it is not clear why we should change the belief.

I conclude then that $c_\psi = c_\phi$: it is the only condition reconcilable with all the principles we hold about such an example. In a nutshell, the argument is simply that overdetermination implies that each event was not necessary, joint determination that each was not sufficient, and in the circumstances both implications are false.

There are three points that should be noted about this argument before I try to meet some objections to it and fill one gap in the argument as stated. The first two points differentiate it from Davidson's argument in 'Mental Events' and the third differentiates it from Lewis's in 'An Argument for the Identity Theory'. The first is that we have in no way assumed that any pair of causally connected token events instantiates a strict law;

[20] For those who favour the logic presented in David Lewis's *Counterfactuals* (Oxford: Blackwell, 1973), the present point can be expressed thus. Let 'O' be the predicate 'occurs' of particular events (analogous to an existence predicate of objects). If overdetermination held, we would have $(\sim Oe_\psi) \mathrel{\Box\!\!\rightarrow} Oe$. Since this is not a vacuously true counterfactual, it implies $\sim Oc_\psi \mathrel{\Diamond\!\!\rightarrow} Oe$. But this is equivalent to $\sim((\sim Oe_\psi) \mathrel{\Box\!\!\rightarrow} \sim Oe)$, that is to the negation of the commonplace that if the pain had not occurred, then the withdrawl would not. Experience has shown that I should emphasize that 'O' is not a predicate true of some events and false of others; it is of course true of *all* events. That is not to say that each particular event is such that it necessarily occurs: we must distinguish the true $\Box \; \forall e \; O(e)$ from the false $\forall e \; \Box \; O(e)$.

Davidson both holds (or held) that, and uses it crucially in his
argument.[21] Second, it does not employ even the apparently
weaker assumption, which would be sufficient for Davidson's
purposes, that any causally related token events are such that
there are physical properties under which they fall in virtue of
which the one causes the other. The third point is simply that
there is no commitment in the above argument to the view that
any particular kinds of physical cause necessarily in general
produce tokens of a given mental state; some arguments that
have been given for identity theories that have turned on causal
considerations have made such assumptions, but this argument
is not one of them.

What of the objections to the argument? I will consider
several.

(i) It may be said that the argument I have given neglects
the possibility of causal relations between c_ϕ and c_ψ themselves.
Let us consider then all the possible cases separately. Anyone
who thinks there is an objection here will of course be allowing
that of two strictly simultaneous events, one may cause the
other, but, though I am sceptical of the possibility and examples
cited in support of it, I shall waive any queries that may raise.
I will, however, take it for granted that the causation relation
is asymmetrical between simultaneous events. There are then
two exclusive cases to consider in discussing this objection, that
of c_ϕ causing c_ψ and that of c_ψ causing c_ϕ. The first of these two
cases really is covered by the argument we have already given.
Even if c_ϕ causes c_ψ, and so it is true (given no overdetermination
of c_ψ and no failsafe mechanisms) that if c_ϕ had not occurred,
then c_ψ would not have occurred, the argument stands. For
still there *is* a causal route from c_ψ to e, one that evidently
cannot pass through c_ϕ given the asymmetry of the causation
relation; and so overdetermination of e remains the case. The
fact that it is true that if c_ϕ had not occurred, then c_ψ would not
have occurred, does not show there is not overdetermination.
We can show this by considering another example. Your pressing a button to light a bonfire electrically may be a signal to
me to put a lighted match to the bonfire at the same time; then
then it is true that if you had not pressed the button, I would

---

[21] See 'Mental Events', p. 99: 'Suppose m, a mental event, caused p, a physical
event; then under some descriptions m and p instantiate a strict law.'

not have put the lighted match to the bonfire, but this cannot show that the resulting fire was not overdetermined.[22] Once we allow causal relations between simultaneous events, if two simultaneous events each cause a third, it is sufficient for over-determination of the third that if *either* one of the two simul-taneous events had not occurred, the third would still have occurred.

In the case of causation of c_ϕ by c_ψ the complaint that there is a gap in the argument presented has more foundation. This is because if c_ψ caused e only via its causation of c_ϕ, as in diagram (A), then it remains true that if c_ψ had not occurred,

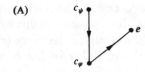

(A)

then e would not have occurred. This evidently in such circum-stances does not contradict the fact that there is a complete physical account of the causal route from c_ϕ to e; on the con-trary, the case requires that that condition is met. So some other argument is needed to deal with this case.

The additional resources for providing such an argument come from empirical suppositions that we mentioned but have not yet exploited about the causation of c_ϕ. We supposed that we had a physical account of the causal antecedents of c_ϕ. By this is meant not the question-begging supposition that there is no nonphysical event that is a cause of c_ϕ, but rather that there are certain physical events prior to c_ϕ of such a kind that we can have empirical reasons for believing that if they had not occurred, then c_ϕ would not have occurred. Now this, it may be objected, is not incompatible with the causation of c_ϕ by c_ψ: an earlier physical event d can both cause c_ϕ and cause c_ψ which also causes c_ϕ, as in diagram (B). But to suppose that in these circumstances the counterfactual 'if c_ψ had not occurred, then e would not have occurred' is true is not to follow the way we

[22] In such examples it may be theoretically helpful to introduce the notion of the overdetermination of an event e relative to a time t: the fire is not overdetermined relative to times prior to your pressing the button, but it is at subsequent times.

(B)

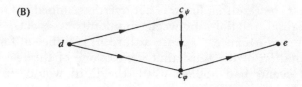

assess the truth value of counterfactuals. Suppose a man flips a switch and causes the light to go on a little time later. The truth of the counterfactual 'if he had not flipped the switch, the light would not have been on a little later' is not altered if this man is President of the local Electric Company, and the only way it could have come about that he did not flip the switch is by his having had to stay at his office to deal with a power crisis that would automatically have triggered emergency supplies and made all the lights in his own house go on. In assessing such counterfactuals we do not allow 'that could only have been because . . .' steps. So in the case represented in diagram (B), it is not an argument for the truth of the counterfactual 'if c_ψ had not occurred, e would not have occurred' that if c_ψ had not occurred, that could only have been because d did not occur, and then e would not have occurred either. Note that this argument, if correct, also tells against the suggestion

(C)

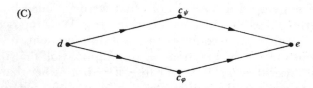

that if the state of affairs were as in diagram (C) then all our suppositions could be reconciled with the distinctness of c_ϕ and c_ψ: for again, these are not circumstances in which it is true that if c_ψ had not occurred, e would not have occurred. Here as earlier in this argument there is appeal to empirical considerations, but it was announced at the start that these would play an essential role in the argument for identity: this could hardly fail to be so, since the identity if true at all is *a posteriori*.

(ii) The second objection is that the argument must be too strong, because it could be used to prove the identity of physical and psychological states ('type–type' identity). But I deny that it could be used to prove such identities. The argument reproduced for states would have to use for *reductio* the supposition that x's being in state S is identical with x's being in state S': this use of the identity sign between gerundive phrases would have to be backed up either with a theory of facts (or states of affairs) or else with a theory of how to eliminate such occurrences. But in any case, the conclusion of the argument will not be an identity between states when this supposition is reduced to absurdity, but only one relativised to x, saying that x's being in state S is identical with x's being in state S'; and the truth of this claim might require no more than that the states S and S' stand in the *realization* relation and not the stricter relation of identity.[23]

(iii) Consider a particular table and the lump of matter of which it consists, and imagine that the table is burned to ashes and energy is released; and suppose that nothing else in the immediate environment is responsible for a release of energy. Now the burning of the table and the burning of the lump of matter do not overdetermine the release of energy; and concerning both the burning of the table and the burning of the lump of matter, we may say that the release of energy would not have taken place without them. Yet for familiar reasons a good case can be made for saying that the table is not identical with the lump of matter. So I am not committing a similar fallacy in the case of events?

What the example shows, according to me, is that it can be true for some substitutions for 'ϕ', 'a', and 'b' that the ϕ-ing of a = the ϕ-ing of b and yet a not be identical with b. In the example, the burning of the table is the very same event as the burning of the lump of matter of which the table consists, and so we do not have a counterexample.

This is an appropriate point at which to make some long overdue remarks on the general views of David Lewis on

---

[23] 'If you allow that x's being in S can be identical with x's being in S' without $S = S'$, then why cannot e_1's *occurring* be identical with e_2's *occurring* without $e_1 = e_2$?' But I have not myself used identity between these gerundive phrases; the argument from the dilemma of overdetermination or joint sufficiency proceeded simply from the assumption (for *reductio*) that the token events e_1 and e_2 themselves are distinct.

psychophysical identity theories.[24] He holds that a common-sense psychology is somewhat like a term-introducing scientific theory: if (roughly) we conjoin all the common-sense platitudes about psychological states, then for any organism, the unique n-tuple of states which satisfies these principles is, definitionally, the sequence of psychological states of which those principles commonsensically spoke. Indeed if T is a theory introducing terms $t_1, \ldots, t_n$, and these are replaced in the theory by new free variables $x_1, \ldots, x_n$ to obtain $T[\bar{x}]$ from $T[\bar{t}]$,[25] in some theories of descriptions

$$(\exists_1 \bar{x}\, T[\bar{x}] \supset T[\bar{t}]) \;\&\; (\sim\!\exists_1 x\, T[\bar{x}] \supset \bar{t} = *)$$

is logically equivalent to

$$\bar{t} = {}_1\bar{x}\, T[\bar{x}]$$

(This will hold in theories of descriptions that have the property, none too plausible for philosophical purposes, that identities between two denotationless terms are counted as true.) It is obvious that there is some overlap between Lewis's view and the detailed claims given earlier about mastery of psychological concepts involving grasp of certain principles: though Lewis does not advert to mastery, some consequences of his view – notably in the case of belief and desire – would be consequences of our earlier contentions about mastery.

One sequence of physical states may satisfy $T[\bar{x}]$ for one creature at one time, and a different sequence may satisfy $T[\bar{x}]$ for another creature at another time. Lewis agrees that this is a possibility, but holds that it is not incompatible with the claim of identity between physical and psychological states. In an earlier, vigorous paper he gives a parallel: 'alignment of slots is identical with being unlocked (for these cylindrical locks).'[26] Here the phrase 'for these locks' may be taken either to go with 'being unlocked' or with 'is identical with'. It is clear from the next page of Lewis's paper, when he writes that his view does not involve 'identity of a defective sort', that he intends the first reading, so let us first consider that. Under this

---

[24] 'Psychophysical and Theoretical Identifications'.
[25] Overlined names and variables denote n-tuples of objects or terms; '$\bar{t} = *$' means that each t_i fails to denote.
[26] 'An Argument for the Identity Theory', *Journal of Philosophy* 63 (1966): 18.

reading, where 'Sx' is a state abstraction operator, might the phrase quoted possibly mean

$Sx(x$ is unlocked and x is of kind $K) = Sx(x$ has its slots aligned and is of kind $K)$?

(Perhaps we should use restricted quantification rather than an extra conjunct specifying the kind: this issue, important elsewhere, is irrelevant to the issues being raised now.) But it is certain that Lewis would not in general accept as true identities of this kind – in particular when the given kind of object does not necessarily have the specified role performed for it by a given physical state, but might have it performed by some other physical state. For Lewis, '$Sx(x$ is unlocked and x is of kind $K)$' is a rigid designator of the state such that an object x is in that state in world w iff x is of kind K in w and is in whatever physical state plays the role of being unlocked *in w*.[27] Now perhaps in the case of a particular lock it *is* plausible that it necessarily has the physical locking mechanism it does; but such an essentialist claim is not plausible for a particular house that can be locked, nor for a particular kind of house; in such cases, amongst which Lewis himself would include psychological and physical states, the analogue of the above identity between states will not be counted as true by Lewis.

Much the most plausible account of the logical form of Lewis's claim would be to regard it as a genuine identity sentence, but now with the identity sign being flanked on one side by a term formed by the application of a functor corresponding to 'unlocked' applied to terms for an object and a time, and on the other by an expression designating a physical state. Thus Lewis's statement that alignment of slots is identical with being unlocked (for these cylindrical locks) would be represented:

$\forall t \, \forall x \, (x$ is a cylindrical lock $\supset F_{\text{unlocked}}(x,t) = Su \, St' \, (u$'s slots are aligned at $t'))$

and analogously we may say that for a given creature x at time t

$F_{\text{pain}}(x,t) = Su \, St' \, (u$ is in brain state B at $t').$

[27] For substantiation of this claim about Lewis, see his additional note at pp. 164–5 of *Materialism and the Mind-Body Problem*, ed. D. M. Rosenthal (Englewood Cliffs, N.J.: Prentice-Hall, 1971).

(The functors 'F_{pain}' and '$F_{unlocked}$' will be in a natural sense nonrigid on Lewis's view.) But if we are sceptical, as of course Lewis is not, that pain and other psychological states necessarily, or indeed actually, have certain characteristic manifestations, we will remain in need of an argument, distinct from Lewis's, for such identities; for the function expressed by 'F_{pain}' from creatures and times to brain states, according to Lewis, picks out at any world what has a certain characteristic kind of manifestation for the given creature at a time with respect to that world. Of course if 'F_{pain}' were reinterpreted so that its output were determined by the realization relation as I defined it in section 1 of this chapter, I could not object to such an identity. Reinterpretation or no, however, it remains that we do not have a true identity sentence linking a *prope name* of the state of being in pain with a proper name of a brain state using the Lewisian apparatus.[28]

I am myself sceptical that in the case of terms like 'pain' there is a nontrivial theory that will play the role of the theory T above in Lewis's account, but I will not argue that case here. Instead I will consider whether, if there were such a theory, common sense psychology would resemble, as Lewis claims that it would, a term-introducing scientific theory. The view of theoretical terms as implicitly defined by the scientific theories by which they are introduced is nothing other than the 'disguised description' view of the meaning of physical magnitude terms that corresponds to the disguised description view of the meaning of proper names; and it is wrong for exactly corresponding reasons. There should be no need to rehearse

[28] We may for curiosity's sake briefly try reading the phrase 'for these locks' as specifying an argument for 'is identical with': a notion 'state S_1 is identical with state S_2 for object x' $(S_1 \overset{x}{=} S_2)$ is then being employed. It is extremely difficult for familiar reasons to make sense of an identity relation that is substantially relativized in the sense that S_1 and S_2 may be identical relative to one object (or possibly object-kind) yet not identical relative to some distinct object (or kind). Is there some restricted analogue for this notion of Leibniz's law? Perhaps the suggestion would be that for any context —— ——, we have that

$S_1 \overset{x}{=} S_2 \supset ($—— x is in S_1 —— iff —— x is in S_2 ——$)$.

But this principle is not true if modal operators are allowed to occur in the context schematically represented by the blank: as we saw, it is easy to think of cases in which we would not maintain that it is necessary that a given role is played in a certain object at a given time by a certain physico-chemically specified state. So we must further restrict the contexts in question: when we do so, we seem to end up with a realization rather than an identity relation.

these here;[29] the main examples are cases in which we clearly say that a man has radically false[30] theoretical beliefs about (and refers to) a certain physical magnitude, rather than more true ones about a magnitude with which he has never been in the right kind of epistemological contract, a kind of contact involving causal connections. (Of course, on the causal picture, certain causal descriptions will always be fulfilled by the reference of a man's terms: but such causal descriptions were given no special status by the view we are considering.) Lewis criticizes Putnam for saying[31] that on the implicit definition view, the terms of a falsified theory would be meaningless: 'if the story theory is unrealized, the theoretical terms are like improper descriptions' and so are not meaningless because we know what they denote with respect to various conceivable nonactual states of affairs. But what Putnam should have said, and no doubt really meant, was that on the implicit definition view, the terms of a falsified theory would be actually *denotation*less: the view in question has the absurd consequence that it is impossible that there should be two successive theories held, both containing some theoretical term *t* that denotes the same thing or magnitude in both theories, the later theory correcting the earlier in important respects about the denotation of *t*. If we are not allowed to say such things, how can we coherently describe the progress of science, or even its possible progress? I am thus not in sympathy with Lewis's claim of parallelism between the cases of psychological term and theoretically introduced terms.[32]

[29] Besides Kripke and Kaplan, see especially Gareth Evans, 'The Causal Theory of Names', *Proceedings of the Aristotelian Society*, suppl. vol. 47 (1973).

[30] Thus Lewis's concession that *near*-realization of the theory may be sufficient ior reference to the state in question ('Psychophysical and Theoretical Identifications', p. 252) is far from enough to cover all the problematic cases. Cf. Franklin's actual view that the electricity discharged in lightning was a *liquid*, and the further false views he could have had without the reference to electricity being destroyed.

[31] 'What Theories Are Not', reprinted in *Mathematics, Matter and Method*, Philosophical Papers, vol. i (Cambridge: CUP, 1975).

[32] In footnote 22 of 'Identity, Necessity and Physicalism' in *Philosophy of Logic*, ed. S. Körner (Oxford: Blackwell, 1976), David Wiggins says against Lewis and on the side of Putnam (in another paper) that `pain cannot be both a neurophysiologically specified brain state and also a functionally specified state: '*If* different particular brain states $B_i, \ldots, B_k$ realize pain in different creatures, and *if* pain is some state in which all these creatures share, then (by transitivity)

4. CONSTRAINTS ON EXPLANATION

Is there an *a priori* argument, an argument of principle, to show that such psychological states as beliefs, desires, and intentions must be physically realized, an argument starting from even more general premises than those used so far? It seems that we can give such an argument to at least the conclusion that beliefs, desires, and intentions must be realized by *some* states distinct from the psychological states themselves: and we seem to have no conception of what these states might be, other than physical states. An initial crude argument to that conclusion might run: 'Beliefs, desires, and intentions explain actions, and explanations must either cite or rest upon *a posteriori* facts: indeed these facts must be *a posteriori* even given the sentence whose truth is to be explained. But we have seen that the principles linking such psychological states as intentions with actions are *a priori*. The psychological states must be realized by states of some other kind, and be subject to the usual *a posteriori* kind of explanation, if attribution of psychological states is to be genuinely explanatory. Beliefs, desires, and intentions could not be "purely mental", whatever that might mean.'

It should be clear that this argument does not involve the fallacy committed in the bad objection to the first reductive view noted in Chapter I, section 2. That objection was a protest against an argument that arrived at a nonidentity by way of illicit substitutions *within* 'it is *a priori* that'; if we construed 'it is *a priori* that' as a predicate of sentences-within-a-language,[33] the fallacy would be analysed as taking as unquoted a quoted occurrence of an expression. But in the present case, under such a construal of 'it is *a priori* that', the arguments proceeds quite legitimately by noting that this *predicate* applies to certain

---

"$B_i \neq B_j$" precludes "B_i = pain and B_j = pain".' I am not endorsing this criticism of Lewis. The ground cited, and the subsequent appeal to the absoluteness of idenity, are decisive against Lewis only if 'the same pain as' is taken as an identity relation. But Lewis could say that 'pain' or 'pain of kind . . .' is an unambiguous *predicate* of brain states, under which several distinct brain states fall. Indeed, this is precisely what Wiggins himself says with great plausibility about 'the same official as': see his *Identity and Spatio-temporal Continuity* (Oxford: Blackwell, 1967), p. 18, the treatment of case (θ). This would, however, admittedly be 'identity of a defective sort' (Lewis, 'An Argument for the Identity Theory', p. 19), something Lewis did not want.

[33] I leave the status of these vague here to avoid being sidetracked.

sentences in a language, whereas it should not do so for genuine explanation to be present. To the argument itself it may be replied: 'A man's ϕ-ing intentionally may have an *a posteriori* psychological explanation because this action results from his desire to ψ and his belief that ϕ-ing is in the circumstances sufficient for ψ-ing; this explanatory source is *a posteriori* because the agent might have had an entirely different goal from ψ in ϕ-ing.' This reply does show that one can reject the argument in question and still maintain the principle that one cannot deduce the beliefs and desires that led him to act from the fact that the agent ϕ'd intentionally by itself. But it would still leave the covering principle of explanation in each particular putative explanation with an *a priori* status. Now why exactly is that objectionable? The origin of our discomfort with such a position seems to be the requirement that an adequate explanation must be such that one can verify the *explanans* statements without verifying the *explanandum*.

Even such a rough statement of a requirement of independent verifiability is not in immediate conflict with the possibility that the covering principle of an explanation is *a priori*: for it does not follow from the fact that it is *a priori* that anything that is $F_1, \ldots, F_n$ is G that one cannot verify that something is $F_1, \ldots, F_n$ without verifying that it is G. (Consider an example in which the F_i are predicates of numbers, and G is a predicate of numbers that it requires a complex proof to show is implied by the conjunction of the F_i.) But the question is whether there is an incompatibility between the requirement of independent verifiability and a stronger property of the covering principle of an explanation. One's immediate inclination is to state the stronger property thus: there would be an incompatibility if the covering principle, that anything that is $F_1, \ldots, F_n$ is G, is required to be known for mastery of at least one of the F_i. But it would be desirable if possible to state the point without using the concept of knowledge. We might try 'in accordance with the principle'; but this 'accord' must be more than just extensional accord in all possible cases, for otherwise we will be back at the problem raised by the mathematical example. Perhaps we can say this: the sense in which knowledge of the principle is required for mastery of at least one of the F_i is that unless someone is prepared to apply the concepts $F_1, \ldots, F_n$

to an object x only in circumstances in which there is for him evidence that that same object is G, we cannot ascribe mastery of all the concepts $F_1, \ldots, F_n$ to him.[34] But we have seen in earlier sections that it *is* plausible that the principles linking belief and desire with action, or intention with action, meet this condition.

Nevertheless a distinction is still being ignored, and an additional argument is needed to show that the covering principle of an explanation cannot be *a priori* even in the strong sense just defined. An objector (call him 'W') might say this: 'I accept the condition that in any genuine explanation it must be possible to verify the singular *explanans* sentences without verifying the *explanandum*. But this is not necessarily excluded by the principle of the explanation being strongly *a priori*, since, for instance, a desire that p is a state such that if the agent is in that state, then if he were to believe that (p iff he χ's), then he would χ. This gives a means of verifying the *explanans* conditions without first verifying the *explanandum* condition in the particular case. *Virtus dormitiva* examples are not explanations, not because their covering principle is *a priori*, but because there is no independent verifiability of their singular *explanans* sentences: and we can find cases in which that last property is altered without making the covering principle *a posteriori*.' This is an interesting position worth some consideration, not least because if correct it would of course have application to the spatial case too. My argument will be that this position just transfers the difficulty to another point, and that the difficulty will in the end be removed only if the covering principles are *a posteriori*.

Let us first consider a more complicated *virtus dormitiva* example in which there is not genuine explanation. Suppose a drug d both puts people to sleep and causes giddiness if taken with alcohol. Let us introduce an expression '$H(\xi)$': any object x is H iff x puts people to sleep and causes giddiness if taken with alcohol. It is not an acceptable explanation of d's putting someone to sleep that it has the property H: even though one

---

[34] Under these conditions, Dummett would say that the most direct method in his sense, of verifying that an object is $F_1, \ldots, F_n$, involves verifying that it is G: cp. *Frege: Philosophy of Language* (London: Duckworth, 1973), pp. 236-9 and elsewhere.

can have evidence that an object is H from the fact that if taken with alcohol, it causes giddiness. It may be replied that this is not conclusive evidence, so there is no parallel with the *a priori* principle of the action case. This is a weak reply since conclusive verification, if it makes sense at all for such E-sentences, requires verification that the agent does indeed act in the way one would expect given both his desires and his beliefs. But the reply can be made more sophisticated: the defender of the position in question ought rather to argue that the difference between the cases is this: while the fact that something would cause giddiness if taken with alcohol is by itself no evidence *at all* that it puts people to sleep, the amassing of a number of counterfactuals of the form 'if the agent were to believe that (iff he χ's, then p), then he would χ' is evidence – though not conclusive – that the agent has the desire that p. So W is still in the field.[35]

But W may remain in the field only because his attacker has mismanaged his case. His attacker can do better by appealing to what we will call *the conjunction restriction* on adequate explanations. The restriction is this. Consider a given covering law L, and consider all the explanations that have L as their covering law. We will suppose for simplicity that each explanation has just one covering law; but the restriction is easily generalizable to the case in which there is more than one. We will also suppose that there is just one singular (if necessary, conjunctive) premise in each such explanation. Let $\{E(\vec{a})\}$ be the set of all singular premises that occur in some explanation that has L as its covering law; let $\{F(\vec{a})\}$ be the set of all sentences that are the *explanandum* sentence of some such explanation. Then the conjunction restriction requires that it is possible, as things actually are, to verify any finite conjunction of sentences in $\{E(\vec{a})\}$ without verifying any sentence in $\{F(\vec{a})\}$. The intuitive rationale for this restriction is as follows. Suppose it were violated: then there is some finite conjunction

---

[35] W might also object to the explanation using H that it could be cut down to one using an *a posteriori* principle. W also needs to take care over the counterfactuals he cites: the truth of such counterfactuals is evidence only if in the altered circumstances the agent does not have different desires. But of course the most direct method of verifying that the agent's desires are not different in the two circumstances involves discovering *which* desires he has.

$E(\vec{x})$ & ... & $E(\vec{z})$ which cannot be verified without verifying some sentence or other in $\{F(\vec{a})\}$. So necessarily if that conjunction is verified, there is some element of $\{F(\vec{a})\}$, $F(\vec{u})$ say, which is verified in the process of verifying the finite conjunction. But now consider the explanation of the conjunction $F(\vec{x})$ & ... & $F(\vec{z})$ & $F(\vec{u})$: the verification of the singular premises of the explanation of this conjunction will have involved the verification of one of the conjunctions that is to be explained. This seems unacceptable.[36] It should be clear that this unacceptability is not avoided by verifying the finite conjunction $E(\vec{x})$ & ... & $E(\vec{z})$ in some other way, for if the conjunction restriction is violated, there will always be *some* element of $\{F(\vec{a})\}$ that is verified when the conjunction is verified, and then there will be no genuine explanation of the conjunction of $F(\vec{x})$ & ... & $F(\vec{z})$ with that element of $\{F(\vec{a})\}$. Thus the fact that 'the' logical form of the crucial part of the conjunction restriction is this:

$$\forall s(s \text{ is a conjunction of elements of } \{E(\vec{a})\} \supset \Diamond (s \text{ is verified}$$
$$\& \sim \exists s'(s' \in \{F(\vec{a})\} \& s' \text{ is verified})))$$

rather than the weaker restriction:

$$\forall s(s \text{ is a conjunction of elements of } \{E(\vec{a})\} \supset \forall s'(s' \in \{F(\vec{a})\} \supset \Diamond (s \text{ is verified } \& s' \text{ is not verified})))$$

does not make its violation any the less objectionable.

It is important not to confuse the conjunction restriction with a stronger restriction, which is not being invoked here; on the stronger principle one is required, for instance, in explaining why a certain combination of sounds is present at a given place at a given time, to explain not only the occurrence of each individual sound, but also the presence of that particular combination. The attacker of W is not committed to that stronger requirement, and can consistently say that sometimes there

---

[36] I am ignoring the difficult problem of providing an account of verification by testimony, for if that is allowed as an objection to the conjunction restriction, it is equally an objection to the claim that what is unacceptable about a *virtus dormitiva* explanation is that one cannot verify the *explanans* without verifying the *explanandum*. This problem is common to all cases and factors out as irrelevant to the difference between acceptable and unacceptable explanations.

will be an explanation of the particular combination of sounds – as when the sounds are produced by several musicians each playing one line of a common score – and sometimes not. The requirement to which the attacker of W is appealing is fully met by the conjunction of the individual explanations of the separate noises heard in a city street. On the weak notion of 'explanation of a conjunction' in question here, the explanation of a conjunction is the conjunction of the explanations of each conjunct.

An example in which the conjunction restriction is violated is this. Suppose we come upon a machine M, perhaps left behind by members of an advanced civilization, which has two display panels. We discover inductively that there is a certain function ϕ such that whenever the numeral for a natural number n is displayed in the first panel, the numeral for $\phi(n)$ (let us call it '$\phi(n)$') is displayed in the second panel. Suppose we introduce the notion 'has the ϕ-property': for an object to have this property is for it to possess the many-track disposition of being such that for any natural number n, if $\bar{n}$ is displayed in its first panel, then $\overline{\phi(n)}$ is displayed in its second panel. Thus it is *a priori* that for any object and for any natural number n, if that object has the ϕ-property and $\bar{n}$ is displayed in its first panel, then $\overline{\phi(n)}$ is displayed in the second panel.

That is *all* that is meant by 'has the ϕ-property'. In particular, to say that something has the ϕ-property is not to hypothesize an underlying mechanism responsible for the presence of the many-track disposition: it is not to say there there is some property P such that it is an *a posteriori* law that any object with P displaying $\bar{n}$ in its first panel will display $\overline{\phi(n)}$ in its second panel. It is merely to assert the presence of the disposition itself. Nevertheless explanation of the presence of $\overline{\phi(n)}$ by the joint presence of $\bar{n}$ and the ϕ-property ought to be acceptable to W. The statement that M has the ϕ-property has infinitely many conditional implications, each of the form 'if $\bar{n}$ were displayed in the first panel, $\overline{\phi(n)}$ would be displayed in the second panel', and many of these conditional implications can be verified independently of any particular truth the presence of the ϕ-property is used to explain. (These implications also have a significant common form, unlike the implications in the case of property H.)

Yet we have a strong intuition that such 'explanations' by means of the ϕ-property are spurious. (This intuition is prior to any high level empirical presumption that physical events have physical causes, for it seems it would still be present even if we had no idea what might be responsible for the behaviour of such machines.) While it is true that the inductive verification of the presence of the ϕ-property can be carried out without verifying the *explanandum* of any particular 'explanation' in which the ϕ-property is invoked, it cannot be carried out independently of *all* the truths the ϕ-property is alleged to explain.

The conjunction restriction on explanation captures this intuition. Let $F_1(M)$ & ... & $F_n(M)$ be the conjunction of all true sentences of the form '$\bar{k}$ is displayed in M's second panel at time t'; let $E(M)$ be the conjunction of the 'explanations' of these conjuncts, if possession of the ϕ-property were by itself adequate explanation for each conjunct. Here the conjunction restriction is violated. The only way of verifying that M has the ϕ-property is to verify that on some occasions what is shown in the display panels has the appropriate form: but of course every piece of such information is already included in the conjunction $F_1(M)$ & ... & $F_n(M)$. The counterfactual implications of 'M has a ϕ-mechanism' do not help, because the verification of any such counterfactual must rest upon the verification of categoricals, and on the view in question the only categoricals that need be true and evidence for such counterfactuals are included in $F_1(M)$ & ... & $F_n(M)$.

I would say the same of the explanation of the actions of a rational agent a. If $\phi_1(a)$ & ... & $\phi_n(a)$ is the conjunction of all sentences 'explained' by an *a priori* principle the antecedent of which mentions the agent's attitudes, then the argument we have just applied to $F_1(M)$ & ... & $F_n(M)$ may be applied to $\phi_1(a)$ & ... & $\phi_n(a)$. For the presence of any one of the attitudes mentioned in the explanation of this conjunction can be verified as things actually are only on the basis of a's intentional behaviour, feelings, or whatever else the *a priori* principle allows intentions to 'explain'; and all the evidence available from this source is already contained in the conjunction $\phi_1(a)$ & ... & $\phi_n(a)$. This general argument applies whatever the other means of verifying the presence of the agent's attitudes W envisages.[37]

Note that the conjunction restriction cannot be reduced to absurdity by arguing that it cannot be applied to a set of *explanandum* sentences that captures everything we believe. The conjunction restriction has no such consequence, because it was explicitly restricted to sets of *explanans* and sets of *explanandum* sentences where these are obtained from explanations using a *given* covering law.

There are some other objections to the conjunction restriction that I will consider. First, it may be said that when the sets $\{E(\vec{a})\}$ and $\{F(\vec{a})\}$ are infinite, violation of the restriction need not be objectionable. Certainly, if the restriction is violated, each verification of a finite conjunction of elements of $\{E(\vec{a})\}$ will involve a verification of some element of $\{F(\vec{a})\}$. But what this means is that if we want to explain the conjunction $F(\vec{x})$ & ... & $F(\vec{z})$ & $F(\vec{u})$ that we have repeatedly fixed upon in our discussion of the restriction, we must then verify the conjunction of elements of $\{E(\vec{a})\}$ in a different way. Provided an infinite stock of ways of verifying any given conjunction of elements of $\{E(\vec{a})\}$ remains, we can always shift the conjunction that is not properly explained elsewhere.

This objection is inapplicable when the set $\{F(\vec{a})\}$ is finite: it is plausible that this is the case in action explanation, since it is plausible that for any given person with a finite life, there will be only finitely many intentional actions he performs. But even in the infinite case the objection is mistaken. If something

---

[37] The general argument for nontrivial realization stated and briefly defended in these few pages places me in disagreement with one of the points in Charles Taylor's 'Reply' in *Explanation in the Behavioural Sciences*, ed. R. Borger and F. Cioffi (Cambridge: CUP, 1970). Taylor there holds that it simply cannot be settled *a priori* whether more basic levels of explanation are mechanistic. If 'mechanistic' is construed to cover every kind of explanation other than those of common sense psychology, the argument of the text insists there must in that sense be a more basic mechanistic level of explanation. 'Mechanistic' may be construed more narrowly, and Taylor asks 'Can we assert today that some version of [psycho-analysis] cannot be more firmly established?' (op. cit., p. 93). Some parts of psychoanalytical explanation make use of the *a priori* principles linking beliefs, desires, and intentions with actions, other parts do not. All I am insisting is that the presence of parts of the latter kind is not an accident if there are to be genuine psychological explanations of an everyday kind of action and psychoanalytical explanation did turn out in some of its parts to be fundamental. (I of course have no disagreement with the other major claims of Taylor's 'Reply', which indeed mesh well with the general position of this section.)

really is the explanation of a state of affairs, it is so independently of the way in which we verify its presence. We cannot find acceptable a situation in which our attempts to explain conform to the following conditional: 'if we had verified the presence of such-and-such state in this object in another way – a way that would have been an entirely legitimate means of verification – then it would no longer be the case that that object's being in that state explains so-and-so.' I am happy to acknowledge that this reply depends upon a realistic conception of explanation.

Second, it may be felt that what I have said about the machine M would exclude cases in which we account for the presence of a many-track disposition by the presence of just one of its tracks. Now presumably someone who offers this objection is not trying to revive explanation by such properties as H that we constructed earlier in this section. He will be wanting to raise the point only when the various dispositions are connected in some way, either by having a common under-lying ground or – if this is intelligible, which is open to serious doubt – by one disposition being the cause of the others. But it is clear that in any case of either of these two kinds the explanation of the presence of the disposition will not violate the conjunction restriction.

How does the conjunction restriction fare in relation to the example of a microscopic theory all the empirically possible evidence for which is stated at the macroscopic level?[38] Certainly if the conjunction restriction were applied to whole theories then such a theory could violate the restriction. All the singular *explanans* sentences in explanation using the theory might be at the micro level, and then these singular sentences could not be verified without verifying some of what the theory is used to explain. So the question is: why apply a requirement to individual laws which is not applied to whole theories? But to that question there is an answer. In any given explanation using a law from the theory, only that law and the singular statements are needed for that explanation to be correct: the rest of the theory is irrelevant to the explanation of this particu-lar phenomenon. The rest of the theory may make plausible the inference to the existence of a law of the kind in this par-

[38] This question was raised by Ernest Sosa.

ticular explanation: but the direction of inference need not be a direction of explanation.[39]

5. FURTHER DEFENCE

Two of the presuppositions of the *a priori* argument for the nontrivial realization of beliefs, desires, and intentions can be questioned. The more radical criticism is provided by what I shall label 'the no-explanation view'; the less radical and more plausible I shall label 'the non-subsumption view'.

The no-explanation view is that an agent's beliefs, desires, and intentions do not explain his actions. The no-explanation view may be combined with various other positions, but the views most plausibly linked with it are these. Explanations must contain *a posteriori* covering laws, a status not possessed by principles linking belief and desire or intentions with actions. The agent's attitudes do indeed *cause* his actions, and that is why the revisionist doctrine that beliefs, desires, and intentions do not explain actions does not impose crippling limitations on what we ordinarily wish to say: we can substitute causal statements as surrogates for the literally false explanatory ones. (There are some questions about reconciling this view with the thesis that causation is a relation between events, but this question of philosophical logic and ontology is not our present concern.)[40] These views would sit naturally too with the doctrines (i) that the predicates of events and states that feature in true 'explains' statements (as opposed to true causal statements) are those that occur in the law that would need to be invoked in a full explanation of the event under the given description, and (ii) that there are no psychophysical laws. For if one holds both these, then beliefs, desires, and intentions cannot explain actions; for if they did there would have to be laws stating that if the agent had certain attitudes and abilities and believed of a certain bodily movement that it would be

[39] The argument of this paragraph does of course exclude a micro theory all the empirically possible evidence for which is at the macro level and which has only one law, where this law is not formed out of several other laws.

[40] The problem is of course that '*a* believes that *p*' does not report the occurrence of an event, but rather that *a* is in a certain state. We do not fully avoid the problem by noting that at least on every occasion on which there is intentional action there is some antecedent genuine event: for we still want it to be true that a person's having a certain belief is something that causes his acting the way he does.

such-and-such kind of event in the circumstances, then there would be a movement of that kind – a psychophysical law. Such is an elaboration and possible source of the no-explanation objection to the argument of the last section.

The non-subsumption view, on the other hand, is that the argument went wrong in supposing that all explanation has to be by subsumption under laws. Action explanation is indeed explanation, but of a different kind from physical explanation: the argument for realization of states that explain when the explanation is by subsumption may perhaps be sound, but action explanation is not an example to which the argument can be applied. A non-subsumption view is a generally recognized option in the literature on action explanation: von Wright sees it as one of the major characteristics of the tradition which rejects assimilation of action explanation to scientific explanation.[41] A typical expression of the attitude is given by Collingwood: 'If, by historical thinking, we already understand how and why Napoleon established his ascendancy in revolutionary France, nothing is added to our understanding of that process by the statement (however ture) that similar things have happened elsewhere.'[42]

The positive theory that underlies the non-subsumption view is normally that to explain an action under the description under which it is intentional is to render it intelligible as something the agent has some reason to do in the circumstances as he (thinks he) sees them. Here there is no talk of laws and subsumption, and there need not be any for the explanation to be good (whatever other arguments there are for saying there must be some in the offing). The holder of the non-subsumption view is in no way specially barred from believing that beliefs, desires, and intentions cause actions, and to avoid irrelevant complications I will assume in the later discussion that he does believe that. But for him what restricts truth-preserving substitutions within contexts governed by '——— explains the fact that . . .' in the case of action explanation is the agent's view of his situation and his operative reasons for acting – nothing about which predicates are in which laws.

[41] Chapter I, 'Two Traditions', of *Explanation and Understanding* (Ithaca: Cornell University Press, 1971).

[42] *The Idea of History* (Oxford: OUP, 1946), p. 223.

I will discuss this non-subsumption view after considering the no-explanation view, since materials we introduce in discussing the latter will be helpful in discussing the former.

We were supposing a no-explanation view according to which attitudes may cause but do not explain actions. Other examples in which we have a true singular causal statement, but in which an explanation statement is false, are based on the prototype of 'The event mentioned on page 3 of today's *Times* caused the event mentioned on page 8 of today's *Times*.' This may encourage the view that it is absurdly weak to maintain that attitudes at most cause and do not explain. While no one would think that the sentence just cited implies that there is a law connecting events mentioned on those two pages of *The Times*, or that it is reasonable if that sentence is true to anticipate a causal connection between the events so mentioned in tomorrow's *Times*, some such expectations do seem to be justified in the action case. It seems much more reasonable to base some expectations about a man's actions tomorrow upon the attitudes that caused him to act today than it does to base analogous expectations on the causal connections between the events mentioned on those two pages of today's *Times*.

It would, however, be quite wrong to think that the defender of the supposed no-explanation view could not easily answer objections flowing from this source. We would expect him to say: 'We have "general knowledge of how persistent various preferences and beliefs are apt to be, and what causes them to grow, alter and decay".[43] Beliefs and desires, or intentions, are constitutively connected with action: if *they* persist, then we should expect them to cause the performance of an action of the type with which they are constitutively connected. Given the general knowledge of the persistence conditions of attitudes that we all have in some rough, unsystematic form, there is no difficulty in accounting for the differences between our action examples and cases in which we know very much less, like the *Times* case, in which we know a true singular causal statement but no explanatory statement.' Thus the imagined no-explanation position is not simply a nonstarter.

The defender of the no-explanation view needs some account of what it is for an action to be intentional under a given description: we know from the examples of Chapter II that causation by, and match with the content of, the intention are far from sufficient. By an 'account' of what it is for an action to be intentional under a given description, I do not necessarily mean some reductive biconditional permitting elimination of 'intentional' in favour of predicates that can be applied in advance of consideration of which actions of an agent are intentional under which descriptions: it would suffice to meet the request to supply a theory that locates the notion of the intentional in relation to other concepts as sophisticated and as deeply involved in the action explanation scheme. (In a similar way Grice's programme may be regarded as helping to exhibit relations between semantic and psychological concepts without an implication that the relevant psychological concepts could be applied without in the pertinent cases use of semantic concepts at some point.) Only if some such account is forthcoming can we avoid the implausible view that the extension of 'intentional under description D' could for all we know vary even though the extension of all other psychological concepts (*including* intention) together with that of 'causes' and 'explains' are fixed.

Be that as it may, the no-explanation view can in any case meet the requirement. For the no-explanation theorist could simply take over the account we offered in the last chapter of the deviant/nondeviant distinction. That is, in terms suggested by this classification of possible positions, the views to be assessed at the moment are those represented in the above diagram by boxes in the lower row generally. We ought not to suppose that all the views falling in the bottom row also fall in the second column: they may fall in the lower left-hand box.

	account of deviance	no account of deviance
attitudes explanatory		
attitudes nonexplanatory	D*	

So: does the box I have labelled 'D*' represent a tenable position?

The question we ought to press on the defender of D* is why he says that certain things that seem to be explanations do not really have that status. Consider the following putative explanation. We have the following premises:

x intends to ϕ at t_0
x's intention to ϕ at t_0 is realized by neural state N
C
K is the kind of movement x believes to be a ϕ-ing in the circumstances

(For brevity I have suppressed a common time reference throughout, and have also omitted the necessary clause that x believes that time t_0 has arrived.) In these sentences, 'N' is to be replaced by a canonical description of a state in the vocabulary of neurophysiology and 'K' by a physical specification of a kind of bodily movement. 'C' is to be replaced by sentences, such as would characterize in the relevant respects the condition of the human body around the appropriate part of the efferent nerve system, whose truth is sufficient for differential explanation of the agent's bodily movement of kind K by the neural state which realizes x's intention to ϕ at t_0. The defender of D* denies that this is a genuine explanation of the agent's ϕ-ing intentionally. What reasons might he have? I will consider two.

The first reason he might express thus: 'The introduction of propositional attitudes is really irrelevant in this alleged explanation. If we completely cut out these together with the realization relation (via which they enter one of the premises), we have then a perfectly good explanation of the occurrence of an event of kind K from the antecedent conditions N and C by means of a purely neurophysiological law. Indeed, such a law gives all the explanatory content of the law in the alleged explanation from propositional attitudes: the law used there is just the neurophysiological law filled out by the use of the realization relation and beliefs about bodily movement types. The extra conditions about realization and differential explanation may be needed in a theory about what makes the event intentional under the given description, but they are not part of the explanation.' But the core explanation this objector sees embedded in the larger alleged explanation, explains the event that is the agent's action under the wrong description: it explains that event as a bodily movement of kind K, but it does not explain it under the other description under which we generally hold it to be explicable, viz. 'movement of the kind the agent believes to be a ϕ-ing in the circumstances'. Moreover, because of the opacity of 'explains' (with respect to predicates, and hence with respect to descriptions with narrow scope), one does not obtain an explanation of an event under description d by adding to an explanation of it under description d' the condition that the events meeting d and d' are identical. (If such a principle did hold, an event explicable under any of its descriptions would be explicable under all of its descriptions.)

Indeed, the double feature, of both containing a physical explanation of a physical event under a physical description and containing psychological vocabulary, is essential if the above form of explanation is to play the role suggested. On the one hand, we have just seen that the presence of the psychological vocabulary is crucial. On the other hand, the purely physical component must be present if the form of explanation is not to be open to objection from requirements similar to the conjunction restriction, from which we argued against W a few pages back. In order to identify an agent's beliefs, desires, and intentions we do indeed need to consider the evidence of all his behaviour (and identifying those attitudes is part of what needs to be done in determining which of this behaviour is intentional under some description); but it is not true that we can verify that the agent x is in state C or in state N in our example only by verifying at least one of the members of the set of all true sentences of the form 'x intentionally ϕ'd [did what he believed to be a ϕ-ing] at t'. I will return to this issue in a more explicit way below.

The second complaint the defender of D* may have against these explanations is that for all that has so far been said, in *any* example in which one state is realized by a second, and an object's being in the second state is explicable by certain laws and initial conditions, then by filling out the explanation by means of the realization relation, we can obtain an explanation as good as those that have been offered in the attack on D* of the object's fulfilment of the first, realized state. But this, the defender of D* will say, is an absurd consequence. For instance, if acid flowing underground would sever a telephone wire, and if the continuity of the wire realizes the direct contact of two people, would it follow that a loss of contact would be explained, under that description, by the flow of acid? That seems wrong, given the presence of some requirement that what explains an event under a description must be specified in terms of the same level as those in that description. Where then is the difference between the action explanations being offered against the defender of D* and the case at which we have just looked?

I suggest that the difference is that in every application of the action explanation scheme, the purely physical law that can be distilled out, in the way that we distilled out the law from N and C to K in our example above, bears a certain uniform relation to an *a priori* principle of a scheme of holistic explanation. In our example, N realizes (for x at t_0) x's intention to ϕ, and K is the physical kind of movement that x believes will fulfil the content of the intention that in fact N realizes. If in the physical law we replace expressions for these physical states by expressions for the psychological states thus related to them, then we obtain a conditional: if x intends to ϕ at t_0 and C obtains, then x executes a bodily movement of a kind he believes to be a ϕ-ing. This is an instantiation (with the detailed physical conditions C replacing the existentially quantified variable 'C') of an *a priori* principle of the scheme of action explanation. It will not of course in general be the *same* purely physical law that is involved in different applications of the action scheme, but each different law will bear the same relation we have just described to the *a priori* principles of the action explanation scheme. In the telephone case, no such principle of a holistic scheme is thus uniformly related to the physical law that is involved in an explanation of the loss of direct contact between a and b under an appropriate physical description. If, contrary to appearances, such a scheme can actually be invented, then I would accept that the event could be explained under the peculiar descriptions of that scheme: but of course 'loss of contact between a and b' is not one of these descriptions. If this suggestion is correct, then only with a theory of what is distinctive of holistic explanation (not necessarily the theory I am offering, of course) can one provide a rationale for the distinction we draw between the two cases. If this account of explanation by attitudes is correct, it seems to be no more than a terminological question whether human action explanation conforms to 'the' deductive-nomological model: though not literally conforming to that model, the explanations given above are closely related to it, and in particular much more closely than on the no-explanation view.

This account of action explanation in fact suggests a generalization to an account of all explanation under non-physical descriptions. The generalization is this. There is a classification of descriptions of events into kinds $K_0, K_1, K_2, \ldots$: these classifications of descriptions are mutually exclusive. These classifications need not be generated by any criterion other than their conformity to the following condition. For descriptions in kind K_0, explanations of events under those descriptions is Hempelian explanation in which the laws contain predicates from amongst those very descriptions themselves.[44] As things actually are, K_0 seems to be the level of physical description. Now suppose we have defined explanation for events under descriptions in K_i and the earlier kinds $K_j (j < i)$. Then a sufficient condition for something to be an explanation of an event e_2 under description ψ_2 from K_{i+1} is that it have this form, where ϕ_1 and ϕ_2 are from some $K_j (j < i + 1)$:

$$\psi_1(e_1)$$
$$\psi_1(e_1) \text{ is realized by } \phi_1(e_1)$$
$$\psi_2(e_2) \text{ is realized by } \phi_2(e_2)$$
$$\underline{C \qquad\qquad\qquad\qquad\qquad}$$
$$\psi_2(e_2)$$

Here $\phi_1(e_1)$ & C must explain the fact that $\phi_2(e_2)$, and there must be some special connection between ψ_1 and ψ_2; in action explanation I have suggested that this is provided by the *a priori*

---

[44] By 'Hempelian explanation' I mean explanation in accordance with the nomological-deductive schema: I do not mean to imply acceptance of the account of lawhood commonly associated with that view of explanation. The associated accounts of lawhood often confuse evidence that a generalization is a law with what it is to be a law.

principles of a scheme of holistic explanation. It is a question for further research what analogous special connections would be present in, for example, sociological or economic explanation. I mention this generalization not just to provide a misty view of the landscape in which my account of action explanation might be located, but to suggest how there might be a uniform account of empirical explanation of which it is an instance.

What of the objections to this account of action explanation? I should first emphasize that I am not saying that one who says that the explanation of an agent's action is that he intended to do so-and-so is *saying* that there are such physical or fundamental realizing descriptions of the agent's intention. Because of the high degree of opacity of 'says that', that is not a consequence. What I am committed to is the view that what he says is true only if there are such realizing descriptions.

An important objection is that explanations of the kind I have offered simply do not always meet the conjunction restriction; in the action case they are explicitly explanations of events under descriptions under which they are intentional, and we cannot verify the presence of an intention in an agent without having verified some other ascription of intentional action. (If we could, our earlier objections to explanation by *a priori* principles would not apply to the action case.)

Certainly the explanations meet a different condition. Their singular premises are not all ones that can be known *a priori* to be true given just the information that the event, characterized by the description under which it is intentional, occurred: nor are the singular premises all ones that can be inductively known (using *a priori* principles) given just a knowledge of all the intentional actions of an agent. Thus we might speak of the explanations as meeting a 'no inference' restriction. Still, what of the objection that they *do* violate the conjunction restriction?

The explanations of the form I propose rest on a level of physical explanation that does *not* violate the conjunction restriction. I want to suggest that the conjunction restriction is plausible for covering law, Hempelian explanation, for whatever is at level K_0 in our hierarchy. Would-be explanations of this kind that violate the conjunction restriction are objectionable, we saw, because in effect they contain *a priori* the facts to be explained.[45] But this objection will not apply to explanation under higher level descriptions if those explanations are of the form I suggested: those explanations cannot simply contain *a priori* the facts of intentional action to be explained, for they contain an *a posteriori* component, and require *a posteriori* laws.

Given this picture, it would be quite wrong to regard the argument that intentions must be nontrivially realized as requiring the addition of some condition that turns an *a priori* principle that covers action explanations into an *a posteriori* one. There is no such *a posteriori* principle common to all cases of explanation of action by the agent's intentions.

It is clear that the physical states that realize an agent's intentions and his ability conditions do not have to be known in order to know that a particular intention explains an event under a description of the form 'event of a kind believed by *a* to be a φ-ing'. Suppose someone accepts this, but maintains that the requirements expressed in the conjunction restriction are satisfactorily met only if to know that some intention so explains an event one must know which physical state realizes it. On pain of contradiction, then, this person will have to hold that 'explains' is ambiguous in physical and psychological explanation if he allows that intentions explanations at all. The contrary view that I have suggested is one that is by no means forced by the data, but is put forward as one that permits us to hold simultaneously (i) that the sense of 'explains' is unified at least to the extent provided by our hierarchy, (ii) that explanations in this sense do not just contain *a priori* the facts to be explained, and (iii) that action explanation is an instance of explanation in this sense.

It may be complained that throughout this discussion I have ignored the role of many *a posteriori* generalizations that we in fact use in employing the action scheme, generalizations relating, for instance, to the conditions of the formation and

---

[45] It may also perhaps be possible to construct an argument that for covering law explanation the no-inference restriction implies the conjunction restriction. One's immediate impression in that there is a gap between the two, for the fact that the conjunction of all the sentences in $\{F(\vec{a})\}$ is not inductively sufficient for some particular statement $\{E(\vec{a})\}$ does not show that it is not necessary. But that is not conclusive; the important question is whether there is an appearance of a gap only because we have not taken into account the full range of states *a priori* connected with the explaining state.

persistence of beliefs and desires. Now so far from denying the existence and important role of such generalizations, I shall actually offer positive arguments for both in the first section of the next chapter. But can such generalizations answer our questions about explanation? Even though we can ascribe intentions only against a background that includes such regularities, those regularities are not part of the explanation of a particular person's intentional action, in the way his possession of an intention and his abilities are. If we want to meet conditions (i)–(iii) of the previous paragraph, more must be involved in action explanation than those background regularities. For how can empirical regularities be what makes citing an intention explanatory, if those empirical regularities are not in the desired way part of the explanation of the agent's action?

A pair of related queries may be raised about the *a priori* argument for nontrivial realization of beliefs, desires, and intentions. The first query asks why the requirement of an *a posteriori* principle of explanation may not be met by an infinite bundle of laws of the form:

For any creature x, if x intends to ϕ and x meets condition C, then x does what he believes to be ϕ-ing in the circumstances

where 'C' is replaced by a physical (in the human case, neurophysiological) condition that in effect expresses internal ability to perform a bodily movement of the kind the agent takes to be a ϕ-ing in the circumstances. Each law in this bundle will be *a posteriori*, and we have no right to complain that it does not supply a single *a posteriori* principle applicable to all instances in which the action explanation scheme is employed, since the proposal I have made does not do that either.

Now it should be noted that if the conjunction restriction on explanation is correct, it is not by itself sufficient for conformity with that restriction that the covering principle of an explanation be *a posteriori*. For the conjunction restriction is violated in any example in which one cannot verify one of the singular premises of the explanation without verifying, as things actually are, one of the elements of the relevant set $\{F(\bar{a})\}$ specified in the statement of the conjunction restriction. But this kind of verification may not be possible even though the covering principle of the explanation is *a posteriori*.

For example, suppose we have a creature for which for all times and for any ϕ, the appropriate physical condition C in the principle from the bundle is always the same. (Examples of this will be somewhat bizarre, but they do not call in doubt the applicability of the action explanation scheme to the creatures they concern.) Since on the bundle view the principles that are explanatory of a creature's actions will contain 'believes', 'desires', or 'intends', the singular premises of the explanation cannot be verified without consideration of the agent's other actions; and in the imagined circumstances this will violate the conjunction restriction. Hence if the conjunction restriction is correct, the bundle theory suggested in this first query cannot cover all the cases.[46]

The difference between the bundle theory and explanations of the form I have proposed is that on the bundle theory explanations containing laws violating the conjunction restriction are not required to rest on explanations containing laws that do not violate the conjunction restriction. My explanations are subject to that requirement. The bundle theorist could of course add a realization relation to his explanations, but it is

---

[46] There is another objection that might be raised against the bundle view. Suppose that one creature x has its intention to ϕ realized by physical state N, and that another creature y, from another galaxy perhaps, has its intention to ϕ realized by a different physical state N'; let x and y both believe that movements of physical kind M will be ϕ-ings; and suppose too that as a matter of physical law N and D lead to an event of kind M whereas N' and D as a matter of physical law prevent any occurrence of an event of kind M. (Rather, the conditions for y's ability to produce a movement of kind M are given by D'.) Now what *a posteriori* law in the bundle can explain x's action of performing what he takes to be a ϕ-ing? We would like to say on the bundle view that the relevant law is obtained from the above scheme by replacing 'C' by some expression for the condition D; but such a 'law' cannot explain anything at all, because it is false. It is falsified in our example when y has the intention to ϕ (realized for him by state N') and is also in state D: of course y cannot then also be in state D', on pain of contradiction, but he is not required to be.

The difficulty with developing this objection is that it cannot be an *a priori* argument to nontrivial realization of all beliefs, desires, and intentions because the problem it adduces can be accommodated thus: the relevant condition substituted for 'C' in the schema on the bundle view may be made dependent upon the way in which the agent's intentions are realized in other states when they *are* so realized, but not when they are not. Such a multiple conditional principle would still be *a posteriori*. The objection has rather to be from the point that the *a posteriori* character of the principle is not by itself sufficient.

hard to see how his view would then differ from the one I
suggested.

The second and related query that might be raised is this.
If we need realization by physical states to make the *a priori*
principles of the action explanation scheme explanatory, do we
not need something analogous in the spatial case to make *its*
a priori principles explanatory? And is there not a threat of
infinite regress in the offing if we require that every physical
state be realized by a distinct physical state?

The important point is that it suffices to meet the conjunction
restriction on explanation that a token experience-event's being
an experience as of its being ϕ can be realized by a token
physical event's having some physical property. (It is unnecessary to insist on identity at this point.) This physical
property may be related by physical laws to its being ϕ at the
place at which the experiencer is located: that is, in the spatial
case we do not need to apply a realization relation to the
E-concepts of the *antecedents* of the *a priori* principles of the
spatial scheme in order to obtain something with premises and
a covering principle that does not violate the conjunction
restriction. It is also to be noted that one of the respects in
which the spatial scheme of explanation is more fundamental
than others is reflected in this fact: the condition that realizes
for a given person at a given time his having an experience of a
certain kind is a condition of a sort that can itself feature as an
E-sentence instantiating one of the conjuncts of the antecedent
of the *a priori* principle of the spatial scheme. The analogous
condition for the action scheme, viz. that the physical conditions that realize a particular person's beliefs and desires are
E-conditions of the action scheme, is not true.

So much by way of criticism and some elaboration of an
alternative to the no-explanation view: I turn now to the non-
subsumption view. This was the view that the argument of the
previous section is flawed by its assumption that all explanation
had to involve subsumption: the non-subsumption view denies
that there has to be subsumption under a law for the citing of
beliefs, desires, and intentions to be explanatory of actions. (The
holder of the non-subsumption view need not deny that laws
are in *some* way involved in all action explanations: his point
is that their presence is not required for the illumination

provided by the explanations.) A basic problem for the non-subsumption theorist is this: if physical explanation and action explanation are so different, how can 'explanation' be univocal in the two cases?

The non-subsumption theorist can offer an answer to this question. He may say that there is no ambiguity in 'explains' because in physical explanation, events are displayed as un-surprising as instances of the way the world works, while in action explanation, events which are actions are displayed as unsurprising given the agent's attitudes, given what he has some reason for doing.[47] Is this an adequate unification?

We would do well at this point to set aside one issue as not central to our problem. When we speak of displaying a particular event as unsurprising, we must not forget that a good case can be made that when there are genuine chance mechanisms in the world, events with very low probabilities can still be explained – explained too under the description under which they are improbable.[48] If this is correct, then 'displaasy unsurprising' had better not mean 'display as likely', on pain of ruling out some physical explanations from the characterization. To bypass this issue, for 'unsurprising' let us substitute 'not ruled out'. (The intent of this modification may be beneficial in the case of action explanation too.)

The central question relates rather to the unity of whatever it is, relative to which the events in the two kinds of explanation are displayed as not ruled out. In the physical case, 'not ruled out given the way the world works' must mean much more than: not ruled out epistemically. It is a familiar point that

---

[47] Some of the phrases in these characterizations are taken from J. McDowell, 'Physicalism and Primitive Denotation: Field on Tarski' (*Erkenntnis* 13 (1978): 131-52), p. 147. I should emphasize both that they are taken from passages McDowell himself notes are gestures in the direction of fuller characterizations, and that by his claims in that paper he is not strictly speaking committed to a non-subsumption view. Non-subsumption and irreducibility are independent. On one hand, one could believe in the irreducibility (by any means) of psychological and semantic notions to the physical, but still hold that action explanation works by subsumption: presumably the subsumption would be subsumption under laws containing psychological vocabulary. On the other hand, one could believe in reducibility, but hold a non-subsumption view of action explanation. For this second combination, however, the ambiguity question would still be pressing.

[48] Cp. Peter Railton, 'A Deductive-Nomological Model of Probabilistic Explanation', *Philosophy of Science* 45 (1978): 206-26.

there are many kinds of example in which the occurrence of one kind of event is not ruled out epistemically given the occurrence of an event of another kind, and this is not sufficient for explanation. (The connection may even be nomological.)

One obvious kind of example is that of two effects of a common cause. It might be that a particular kind of sore throat and of headache a little later are each caused by (and only by) a certain cold virus. Given the occurrence of such a sore throat, a headache later is not only not ruled out, it is to be expected, and the principle by which it is to be expected can be as well confirmed as anything ever can be: but obviously the occurrence of the sore throat does not explain the occurrence of the headache.[49] So what matters is that the event not be ruled out given the causal laws. There are now two ways the arguments may be developed, according to whether it is thought that physical explanation just is definitionally a certain kind of deduction from causal laws, or whether it is thought that the relevant deduction from causal laws has some independently specifiable property which makes it the appropriate model for physical explanation. Suppose we take the former stance. Then the unification offered in effect says that: in the physical case, events are displayed as not excluded given the causal laws (and initial conditions), and in the action case as not excluded given the agent's attitudes. In both cases the question is: what unifies causal laws and the agent's attitudes as that relative to which events are not excluded? What we would so like to say is that in each case these are what *explain* events under the descriptions in question. But that could be said even if 'explains' were not univocal. If an account is faced with the question of whether according to it 'explains' is ambiguous, the question

---

[49] It also does not cause the headache. Can one use this to avoid the conclusion to which I am driving, that one needs to employ the concept of causal necessity in explaining physical explanation? In particular, could one avoid it if one held a counterfactual theory of causation plus a theory of counterfactuals that does not make appeal, direct or indirect, to the notion of causal laws? Even then it is arguable that one would need to use the notion of causal possibility in specifying *which* counterfactuals have to be true. First, the counterfactuals have to hold not just for all actual instances, but for all causally possible instances. Second, it seems possible to construct devious examples in which the counterfactuals corresponding to a generalization that is not a law are true, and it appears these cases have to be excluded by requiring that the counterfactuals be true even when certain causally possible conditions are added to their antecedents.

is not resolved in its favour by suggesting a property common to the two cases specified using the very word 'explains'. Similarly, suppose we take the second stance about physical explanation. Then general question just becomes this: what *is* the independently specifiable property which both explanation by causal laws and explanation of human action share?

That is the main question I would raise for the non-subsumption view. It is also a temptation for one critical of the non-subsumption view as a criticism of the argument of the last section to maintain further that causation and rationalization by attitudes are not sufficient for explanation. And it is hard not to have some sympathy for this view. In our newspaper example, for instance, we could invent the concept of one event being an 'earlierpagination' of another: one event stands in this relation to another if the first is mentioned in the same issue of some newspaper on an earlier page than the second. Are causation and earlierpagination sufficient for explanation, and if not, why should causation and rationalization be so? – This is a good question but it is a mistake to take the problem it raises as one for the non-subsumption view. The non-subsumption theorist can simply take over what I myself said in Chapter I about holistic explanation in order to distinguish the two cases: so either he has an answer to the criticism, or that account in Chapter I is wrong. Indeed the putative criticism is a red herring: the problem at present is not what is distinctive of action explanation, but why whatever is distinctive of it is sufficient to make it *explanation*.

My own tentative answer to the ambiguity question would appeal to the hierarchy we discussed earlier. The suggestion would be that for a kind of explanation to be explanation in the same sense in which physical explanation is explanation, it is a necessary condition that the given kind of explanation occur somewhere in the hierarchy based on K_0, K_1, K_2, . . . of a few paragraphs back. Such an answer is only programmatic, and it must be filled out with an account of the restrictions that limit higher level explanations – why, for example, 'earlierpagination' is not allowed but rationalization is. I will not undertake to implement this programme here, for any convincing answer must look not only at action explanation but also biological, sociological, economic, and all kinds of higher-level explanation. My point here is just that the hierarchy account leaves room for the development of an answer to the ambiguity question.

In some respects the differences between the non-subsumption theorist I imagine and the position I have suggested are small. The point is not just that the non-subsumption theorist's positive account of action explanation is something I can agree to, and incorporate at some level in the hierarchy, though that is true. It is also that the *a priori* principles of the action scheme relate only intentions to actions. Nothing I have said implies one can predict actions on the basis of the agent's attitudes other than his intentions, nor in particular just on the basis of his beliefs, desires, and emotions; nor does it imply that there must be *a posteriori* laws of human nature stated solely at the psychological level. In so far as the rejection of the need for such principles for the possibility of action explanation is part of the motivation for the non-subsumption view, it is one that I share.

The phenomenon of knowledge without observation has not featured in any of the positive parts of the above account of action explanation. Professor Anscombe has however placed some weight on the claim that 'the class of intentional actions is a subclass of' 'the class of things known without observation'.[50] Care is needed in formulation here, since 'things known' are specified by complete sentences, but intentional actions are specified by descriptions of particular (token) events. The claim, schematically, seems to be that if someone ϕ's intentionally, he knows without observation that he is ϕ-ing.[51] Let us call this claim '*A*'. *A* does not seem to be true in the general case. One may operate a remotely controlled device and not know that one is ϕ-ing (e.g., making the toy plane bank to the left) even though one intends to and succeeds. One need not even believe one is ϕ-ing if the device is unreliable, but this does not seem to me to show the ϕ-ing not to be intentional in those cases in which ϕ-ing does result (via a nondeviant chain, it should go without saying). Of course there will be other

---

[50] *Intention* (Oxford: Blackwell, 1957), p. 14. The two quoted phrases occur in the reverse order in her text, separated by other matter, but what she writes clearly implies the formulation I give.

[51] The last four lines of p. 50 and other passages seem to require this reading.

descriptions under which such an event is intentional, if only 'performing a bodily movement of a kind believed sufficient to make the controlled object do so-and-so if the device works'; but Professor Anscombe appears to make the claim for any description under which the event is intentional.

A weaker claim would be that anyone who ϕ's intentionally knows that he acts (or is aiming to act) with that intention. (Even if true, this principle would not of course help towards a noncircular analysis of intention, but it could still be a distinctive feature of intentions.) A speculative objection to this claim is that a neurophysiologist might, as we noted, succeed in blocking the causal route to the agent's beliefs from the essential initiating events, of which Pears wrote. But a conclusive objection to the weaker claim is that it entails that any creature with intentions, say a cat in pursuit of a bird, has the concept of intention and ascribes intentions to itself. More generally, we may say that explanation by reasons is a species of holistic explanation, and when in this area the phenomenon of knowledge without observation arises, its status as knowledge has the same explanation as it does elsewhere, viz. that supplied by the causal generation of the beliefs together with an adequate causal account of knowledge.

We need to ask why the grounds Professor Anscombe had, that would encourage one to hold A, do not really carry one all the way to A itself. She notes that 'it is an error to try and push what is known by being the content of intention back and back';[52] this view she supports by an example in which some perceived object is kept level by executing a pumping movement with the arm. The downward movement of the arm is intentional under the description 'keeping the object level' but not (for most of us) under the description 'lowering one's arm at the rate at which it would naturally fall', a description under which each downward movement in fact falls. There is nothing in this example that could not be granted by someone who desnies A: it would present a difficulty for him only if he held that what was known without observation in every case of intentional action was at the same level, concerned with bodily-movement predicates (or even earlier). But there is no

[52] *Intention*, p. 53.

need for the denier of A to make that assumption: it seems it could only rest on the suspect view that if a piece of knowledge of a certain kind is sometimes inferential, it always is. For instance, in a standard case, the denier of A can consistently allow that someone writing on the blackboard with her eyes shut can know without observation that she is doing so.

Finally I will try to fill a lacuna in one argument sometimes offered for a causal theory of action. The argument is that in giving conditions for intentional action we need to turn the 'and' in 'he did it and he had appropriate reasons' into a 'because', and a causal theory accounts for the need for this 'because'.[53] This is certainly a virtue of the causal theory, but as an argument it is incomplete; for one needs to show that other, noncausal, ways of accounting for the 'because' are defective. After all, 'because' does not always signal a causal connection. A rival account might take the notion of 'ϕ-ing intentionally' as primitive, and then appeal to an *a priori* principle: 'Someone ϕ's intentionally iff he intends to ϕ, believes the moment is ripe, and is able to ϕ intentionally', to explain the 'because'. This would make the 'because' like that in: 'He's a bachelor because he's a man and unmarried.' (Ability in the *a priori* principle offered by this theorist will need a wide construal.)

Such a theory is inadequate on semantic grounds. 'To ϕ intentionally' and 'to have the intention to ϕ' are not semantically unrelated. A causal theory offers one clear suggestion about the connection: one ϕ's intentionally whenever an intention to ϕ differentially explains a bodily movement believed to be a ϕ-ing. On a noncausal theory containing the components we just suggested, the semantic connection is left quite obscure: no account of what it is to have an intention is given when one is not acting intentionally. (It is not sufficient for me now to have the intention to ϕ in two weeks' time that I have the disposition to ϕ intentionally then: that is consistent with my not yet having formed the intention.) This argument does not presuppose that either 'intention' or 'acting intentionally' be regarded as fundamental, but only that a sufficiently close connection be exhibited between them.

[53] D. Davidson, 'Actions, Reasons and Causes', *Journal of Philosophy* 60 (1963), 685–700, sections III, IV.

6. INDEXICALITY AND POINTS OF VIEW

I turn now to consider the sources of the bafflement and even repugnance many people feel when confronted with physicalist theses. My aim is not at all to discredit the sources of these intuitions, but rather to show that we can accept the thought behind some of them without rejecting the weak physicalist theses I have already suggested. We can identify two, perhaps three sources of bafflement.

A first source is this. The truth values of the sentences of physics and the physical sciences generally can be investigated by intelligent beings with quite various and possibly radically different kinds of sensory apparatus: the truths of these sciences are available to many different standpoints. On the other hand, for any organism which has conscious states, 'there is something it is like to *be* that organism – something it is like *for* the organism.'[54] If certain states just *are* ways it may be like to be an organism of a certain kind (and certain kinds of bodily pain may be said to be just such states), then it seems absurd to suggest that such states can be investigated by a science accessible to creatures who may be unable to experience them.'Any shift to greater objectivity – that is, less attachment to a specific viewpoint – does not take us nearer to the real nature of the phenomenon: it takes us farther away from it.'[55]

If a predicate ψ is intelligible only from a certain viewpoint in Nagel's sense, then must ψ be irreducible to predicates of physics? Clearly we need here a distinction between semantic and nomological reducibility. A predicate ψ is semantically reducible to a possibly complex predicate ϕ if one who knows that ψ and ϕ are coextensive, and understands ϕ, is in a position to know everything known to one who understands ψ. ψ is nomologically reducible to ϕ if it is causally necessary that all and only ϕ's are ψ's. If ψ is intelligible only from a certain viewpoint in Nagel's sense, then clearly ψ is semantically irreducible to predicates of the physical sciences. We ought not, though, to rule out the possibility that it is nomologically reducible to them: this would not conflict with the fact that

[54] Thomas Nagel, 'What is it Like to be a Bat?' p. 436.
[55] Ibid., p. 445.

ψ is intelligible only from a certain viewpoint, since nomological reductions need not be a means of conveying understanding.

What about the converse? Is semantic irreducibility sufficient for a predicate to be intelligible only from a certain viewpoint? It may be suggested that belief is a counterexample to such sufficiency: for certainly beings of very different constitutions and possessed of very different kinds of experience can succeed knowingly in attributing beliefs to each other, to us, and to others of yet different constitutions. But I am not convinced that *this* is a counterexample to sufficiency, for I am not convinced that belief is irreducible.

This may sound outrageous: how can I claim that belief is reducible when much of Chapter I of this essay was devoted to arguing for those irreducibility principles? The answer is that there is a distinction to be drawn. What was argued in section 3 of Chapter I was that there was no physicalistic reduction of belief that does not appeal to the *a priori* principles and the intertemporal constraints upon the application of the E-concepts of the scheme. There was no objection to (though also no confirmation of) a reduction that succeeds indirectly in appealing to them.

There should be no need to give an exposition of the form of such a reduction, for it has been given with great clarity by Lewis and Field.[56] Suppose (perhaps *per impossibile*) we can fully specify as a set of principles the *a priori* relations that must hold between sensory inputs, belief, desire, intention, and action, both at a given time and over time. (We thus incorporate the intertemporal constraints on the application of the E-concepts.) Imagine this set of principles written out with a different indexed schematic letter replacing each expression for a psychological state, like 'believes'. Clearly we can define the notion of a temporal succession of sequences of states fulfilling this set of principles, and using this notion we can offer a higher order definition of any one of the psychological states mentioned in our original set of principles. The technical details are given in Field's paper. I am not endorsing such a position (cp. the end of Chapter I): what matters for us here is that the possi-

[56] Lewis, 'Psychophysical and Theoretical Identification'; H. Field, 'Mental Representation', *Erkenntnis* 13 (1978): 9-61.

bility of such a position shows that it is not obvious that belief is a counterexample to the claim that semantic irreducibility implies intelligibility from certain standpoints only. Indeed the force of the Lewis–Field suggestion lies not only in its suggested reduction of psychological states: it also makes it plausible that in so far as the notion of belief is accessible from different points of view, the principles governing it must be statable in the schematic form their construction employs. That is, either the notion has such a reduction or it is not accessible from all standpoints.

More generally, if a predicate ψ is semantically irreducible to the predicates of the physical sciences, and the states of affairs investigated in the physical sciences are the *only* ones accessible from all viewpoints, then ψ must be intelligible (if at all) only from certain viewpoints.

Our original question was whether the fact, if it is one, that certain predicates are intelligible only from a certain viewpoint, is incompatible with the physicalist doctrines I have already defended. Now the doctrines I have defended do not imply that psychological predicates are either semantically or nomologically reducible to open sentences of the physical sciences. I argued only for a token identity thesis, a realization doctrine, a principle of physical embedding, and took supervenience of mental on physical predicates to be plausible. The first of these doctrines is ontological, the second causal, the third concerns an explanatory asymmetry, and the fourth concerns a non-translational relation between vocabularies. None implies there are not predicates of events and states that are intelligible only from a particular kind of viewpoint. 'Is ascribable only from a certain viewpoint' is a predicate of predicates, not of the token events which are – in the sense of identity – sums of events satisfying some predicate of physics.[57] This makes me not a physicalist with respect to properties.

There is however a second interesting statement of the anti-physicalist intuition that has been offered by Thomas Nagel, and which if valid would not so clearly be innocent of onto-logical implications that contradict those weak physicalist

---

[57] In the article last cited, Nagel notes the possibility of essentially the position outlined in this paragraph and remarks 'we may have evidence for the truth of something we do not really understand'.

theses.[58] Suppose I am given as complete a description as you please of the world without using any token-reflexive (indexical) expressions. Such a description can include a specification of each person's thoughts, intentions, and emotions as well as descriptions of the states of inanimate objects: there is no restriction on the kind of predicates that may be employed, as long as they are nonindexical. Now however complete we make this description, 'there seems to remain one thing which I cannot say in this fashion – namely which of the various persons in the world *I* am'.[59] No addition of nonindexically presented information – though for any true sentence of a physical science, we include it – will entail what is nevertheless true, viz. that I am C. Peacocke.

All that seems to me indisputably true. But a first observation to be made upon the failure of this entailment is that it seems to be a property of indexical expressions generally. For example, form as complete a nonindexical specification of the world as you please, it will not follow that *this* country is England. Given the information that this country is uniquely *F*, then some nonindexical description of the world that states that England is uniquely *F* will allow us to infer that this country is England; but without some such indexical premise, we could not reach such a conclusion from nonindexical information alone. But none of this inclines us to deny that 'this country' as uttered by someone on a particular occasion in England refers to the very same object as does the nonindexical 'England'. (Pick a definite description not containing indexicals to replace 'England' if you think with Burge that on a particular occasion of utterance 'England' functions like as demonstrative.[60]) Exactly similar points could be made with 'here' and places or with 'now' and times. The general point here I will label 'the irreducibility of indexical reference'.

It is a major desideratum in both semantics and the philosophy of mind to have a theory of indexical as opposed to nonindexical reference that demonstrably has the consequence that the former is irreducible to the latter: I will not discuss the form of such a theory further in this work, but will confine

[58] 'Physicalism', *Philosophical Review* 72 (1965): 354-6.
[59] Ibid., p. 355.
[60] 'Reference and Proper Names', *Journal of Philosophy* 70 (1973): 425-39.

myself to noting the existence of one extremely striking connection that is relevant to the role of indexical reference in anti-physicalist thought. Thomas Nagel has observed that a number of philosophical debates have a common form, being concerned with an apparent conflict between an objective and a subjective viewpoint on a given issue:[61] amongst others, he cites issues of personal identity, the mind–body problem, and problems in the philosophy of space and time, as having the features with which he is concerned. One striking phenomenon is that whenever we have a thought expressed using indexicals, this thought is one that falls on the subjective side of the subjective/objective distinction: the first person pronoun is naturally used in the expression of the subjective standpoint on questions of the self, 'here' and 'now' are associated with a subjective viewpoint in space and time (with 'this F' perhaps locating an object from such a subjective standpoint). In some of these cases the use of indexical reference seems essential to the expression of a subjective viewpoint. A further requirement on a theory of indexical reference and on a theory of the subjective/objective distinction is that it should explain the naturalness of using indexicals to express a subjective point of view. If what is characteristic of indexicals is that they do not contain a recognitional component (in other words, competent use and understanding of them does not[62] involve the possession on the part of the speaker of a given capacity for recognizing a particular object), then the connection we have noted might incline us to see the exercise of capacities for recognizing particular objects as (one component) of what produces a natural expression of an objective attitude. It is as if there are two categories of truths available to us: there are those we can learn directly without exercising a capacity for recognizing a particular object, and there are those that are not, and only the latter can be expressed from a subjective point of view in Nagel's sense. I take it that this is a subject on which a great deal of further thought and more precise formulations of distinctions are required.

[61] 'Subjective and Objective', mimeo circulated December 1975.

[62] Excepting of course when there are proper names embedded in a complex F in *that F*.

It may be protested that there is a source of an anti-physicalist intuition that is not properly captured by the formulation in terms of indexicals, even in areas in which indexicals are essential to the expression of the subjective point of view. It might be said that what the indexical formulation failed to capture was what Nagel was gesturing at when he wrote that his experiences are underivatively his, and only derivatively his body's by virtue of their causal connections.[63] It is not absolutely clear that we can give a relevant sense to 'derivative' here if we defend (as Nagel also did) the token–token form of identity theory: in what sense are mental events only derivatively my body's if they are identical with token neurophysiological events in the matter of my brain? (Perhaps they are only 'derivative' under a description, and that would not provide any objection to the physicalist claims.) But in any case it seems that we *do* have some analogue of the distinction between the derivative and the underivative in other areas in which there is indexical reference. We might say that in just the sense that these experiences are underivatively mine, and only derivatively associated with a given body, a certain perspective is underivatively here, and only derivatively associated with a given place. (The contingency of the association of perspectives and places, depending on the way the world is at various places, cannot undermine this parallel, for it is also true that I might have been having experiences of a different kind from those that I actually am having.) One seems to need no exercise of a recognitional capacity or *a posteriori* checking that certain relations hold between them, to know that this perspective is here, any more than to know that these experiences are mine. There may be differences in respect of corrigibility between the cases, but our concern was whether there was a corresponding distinction between the derivative and the underivative.

These sources of dissatisfaction with physicalism of the weak kind I have offered, so subtly isolated by Nagel, need not then tell against it. Nagel is also clearly right that these sources of dissatisfaction are not met by postulation of a new entity: all the same problems will arise for it too. But it is also clear that not all cases in which we wish to speak of a subjective standpoint

---

[63] 'Physicalism', pp. 353–4.

are traceable to indexicality: and in particular the subjective aspect of conscious states cannot be traced to indexicality. There seems to be no significant sense in which 'is in pain at time t' is an indexical predicate. The most, then, that these points about indexical reference can show is that there is no necessary connection in general between a subjective viewpoint and nonphysical objects.

IV
INTERPRETATION

1. APPLYING A SCHEME

I now turn to what I shall label 'quasi-reductions'. To specify a quasi-reduction for a given scheme of holistic explanation ('H.E.') is to specify some concept Q and some method M applicable to a set of truths stated using Q that meet the following conditions:

(i) Q cannot be possessed by someone with no grasp whatsoever of the given scheme of H.E.;

(ii) one can know that an object is Q without knowing which detailed E-concepts of the scheme apply to it;

(iii) M takes one from a set of truths stated using the concept Q but not using detailed applications of the E-concepts of that scheme, to a particular set of detailed applications of the E-concepts of the given scheme. (Here we may speak of the 'output' of the method M for that set of truths.)

Requirement (iii) does not of course demand that Q be applicable in advance of knowledge of the *a priori* principles of the scheme (on the contrary, requirement (i) militates against that). The interest of the notion of a quasi-reduction lies naturally in the fact that if such a quasi-reduction can be supplied for a scheme of H.E., we thereby have a means by which someone without prior knowledge of the detailed application of its E-concepts to particular objects may come to know truths stated using them; but using such a method does not mean that he is necessarily able to reduce the E-concepts to other concepts which can be understood independently of that scheme of H.E.: a quasi-reduction is not a reduction. (The method M is not precluded from also making use of truths not employing the concepts Q, provided these truths do not employ detailed applications of the E-concepts. of the scheme in question.)

Thus it may be alleged that the concept of holding a sentence true and Davidson's radical interpretation procedure[1] function

---

[1] See 'Radical Interpretation', *Dialectica* 27 (1973): 309–23; 'On the Very Idea of a Conceptual Scheme', *APA Proceedings and Addresses 1973–4*; 'Belief and the

as the concept Q and the method M respectively of a quasi-reduction for some fragment of the scheme of action explanation in terms of beliefs, desires, and sentence senses. The same status might be attributed to a preference ordering and Ramsey's method[2] of arriving at an assignment of subjective probabilities and utilities from that ordering. Given the structure and cases of holistic explanation that we have already discerned, it can hardly fail to be true that there is some interesting conclusion available from further thought on quasi-reductions. For the following cases exhaust the possibilities. Either there is some reason that a quasi-reduction must be available for any system of H.E., in which case one must see why it must and what the quasi-reduction might be in the spatial case; or a quasi-reduction is available in the action and propositional attitude cases and not in the spatial case, and if so the ground of this difference needs to be discovered; or else an account of how a scheme of H.E. is applied in no way requires that a quasi-reduction be available, and this may lead to scepticism about such quasi-reductions as have been proposed.

I shall argue for that last alternative. Nevertheless it is a fair question to put to me why anyone should ever have thought that a quasi-reduction *ought* to be available for any given scheme of H.E. I said that a quasi-reduction at least shared with a reduction the property that if one were given, it would supply a means by which someone without prior knowledge of the detailed application of the E-concepts of a scheme could come to know truths stated using them. But the truth of the irreducibility principles shows that any presumption in favour of reduction is incorrect, and why should anyone want a surrogate for it? Clearly, since I shall be arguing against the possibility of a quasi-reduction in the action and spatial schemes, I do not think an answer to this question can be given that *should* compel us to demand a quasi-reduction: but it is still reasonable to ask me to cite considerations that could intelligibly

---

Basis of Meaning', *Synthèse* 27 (1974): 309–24; and 'Thought and Talk' in *Mind and Language: Wolfson College Lectures 1974*, ed. S. Guttenplan (Oxford: Clarendon Press, 1975), pp. 7–23.

[2] See 'Truth and Probability', esp. section (3), in his *The Foundations of Mathematics and Other Logical Essays* (London: Routledge, 1931).

move someone to make the demand, if the arguments against the demand are not to be arguments against a straw man.

What motivates those who ask for a quasi-reduction is the fear that there is an indirect circularity in the application of the E-concepts of a scheme. Consider the spatial case. Suppose a man asks what would be evidence that it will be ϕ (that it will rain, say) in the near future at a given nearby place. The answer 'If you go there, and your perceptual system is working, you will have an experience as of its raining' helps the questioner only if he knows where he is relative to the place in question, he is able to check that he is at the correct intermediate places on his route, and so forth. This is just a restatement of the intuition that we expressed at the start of Chapter I, to the effect that the experience-kinds to be expected given the obtaining of a particular E-truth in the spatial scheme are not independent of which other E-sentences are true. The quasi-reductionist then sees the threat of a circularity because if one is not able to apply the E-concepts *at all*, then one will not know what to take as evidence for a given E-sentence. The quasi-reduction is intended by its proponent to free one from this difficulty. Exactly similar considerations apply in the action case: the evidence that a person has a given belief will be its consequences in combination with his other beliefs and desires. If we are not able to apply the E-concepts at all, we will not be justified in taking one thing rather than another as evidence of a particular belief or desire.

The structure of the argument in this section will be as follows. First we will consider a simple example and see how the spatial and (in a sense to be explained) the prespatial schemes of H.E. come to be applied without the use of a quasi-reduction, and draw a few simple lessons. We will then be in a position to note that all these points and lessons apply *pari passu* to the attribution of beliefs, desires, and meanings. The materials will then be available for showing that no conclusion favourable to the possibility of quasi-reduction follows from, for instance, the true observation that one can know that a man holds a sentence to be true without knowing what it means on his lips. The considerations that suggest such an inference to be a *non sequitur* lead to the view that the only possibility for a quasi-reduction must be in an integrated theory of interpretation and decision, and I will conclude by outlining one form such a theory might take and criticizing it.

It is clear that any sequence of experiences whatever could be regarded as produced by tracing a path in a space, in the severely limited sense that for any sequence of experiences whatever, we could envisage some assignment of features at various times to places in a space, and a route through that space, that would yield those experiences. But it is also equally clear that very many such sequences of experiences provide in themselves absolutely no basis for saying that a change in experience results from a change of place by the experiencer rather than a change at a place. (Of course, the same point is true for constancy of experience.) While this second observation shows that the applicability of the spatial scheme of H.E. may be restricted to just some of the allegedly possible[3] sequences of experiences (for there is no other basis for application of a scheme than experience itself), the first observation serves as a reminder that in the nature of the case one can never conclusively establish that a change or persistence in experience is to be explained by successive properties of a single place as opposed to successive properties of different places.

An easy way of seeing the kind of basis experience can supply in itself for drawing the distinction between change of place and change at a place is by constructing a very simple example.[4] For a reason to be given after the details of the example, but which may emerge during its statement, I will in this example speak not of space and the places comprising it, but of prespace and the preplaces comprising it. Let us then imagine a prespace with (for our purposes) just four preplaces, labelled 1 to 4, and ordered as in the diagram below. These preplaces may display

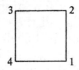

[3] Of course, if Strawson's central argument in *The Bounds of Sense* (London: Methuen, 1966), pp. 97–112 is correct, then not all these apparently possible sequences are genuinely possible courses of experience. I will not pursue this fascinating issue here.

[4] The example is given only to show how such a basis can be applied: it is obvious that the real world is infinitely more complex, our knowledge of it much more fragmentary, than in this example.

observable qualities F, G, . . . , L which are taken to be exclusive and need not be taken to be intrinsically spatial in the way some features available to sight and touch are. If one wishes to avoid any hint of discontinuous motion in this prespace, one may suppose either (a) that these qualities admit of variation in intensity, being most intense at the 'centres' 1, 2, 3, and 4, and fading at points between them, or (b) contingently the qualities, perhaps sounds, have sharp boundaries. (In both cases, it may be said that there are really 'more' preplaces than 1–4, but in the latter case, given the way things happen to be, and given only the descriptive resources of expressions for F, . . . , L, there would be no way of discriminating any other preplace from all of 1–4.)

A segment of the history of such a world is given in the displayed table below, the left to right ordering of entries on a given row representing the temporal ordering of occurrences of a quality at a given preplace, while occurrences represented in the same column are simultaneous. The line aa' represents a possible experiential route through this world. In this world,

time ⟶

	t_0			t_1				t_2		t_3 t_4 t_5

```
        t0                    t1                              t2            t3 t4 t5

1 ᵅF̶ G̶ H̶ F̶ G H F G H F G H F G H F G H F G H F G H F G H F

2 G K G K G̶ K̶ G̶ K̶ G̶ K̶ G K G K G K G K G K G K G K G̶ᵅ'K̶ G K

3 J F J F J F J F J F F̶ F̶ F F F J F J F F̶ J̶ K̶ J F J F

4 G H L G H L G H L G H L G H L G̶ H̶ L̶ G̶ H̶ L G H L G̶ H L G
                                                      β
```

regularity is provided by the cycles of qualities at each preplace; but in the use to be made of the example there is nothing that would prevent secular alteration in these patterns.

It seems that the sequence of experiences determined by aa' is one which would in itself contain the materials for drawing the various distinctions we are actually able to draw which involve the concept of location. It is plausible that someone with such a course of experience would by time t_2 have in his by then relatively small class of theories of the world the true description of the world, and it seems obvious that it is possession of a particular empirical theory of regularity that would permit him to conclude at t_5, for instance, that at t_4 he had moved to preplace 2 rather than moving in the other direction to 4 or staying put at 3. For if he had followed route $\alpha\beta$ and been at preplace 4 at t_4 he could have experienced only F, H, or G (at preplaces 3, 4, or 1 respectively) at the next time t_5, and not K as he actually does. Once the theory is going, we can also allow for hallucinations.[5] All this is in simplified form my answer to the question of how we can avoid the circularity that motivated the demand for a quasi-reduction without actually having a quasi-reduction.

I have written (and shall continue to write) as if there were an ontogenetic stage at which an experiencer views himself as having experiences and raises the question of the explanation, if any, of them; and this, it may be said, is simply to beg the question against the Kant–Strawson view that experience can only be construed as such, and so is only possible at all, for a being equipped at least with the idea of an objective world and, if such a world has to be spatial, of a route through it. But in fact that fundamental question is not being begged: it does not matter for present purposes if the notion of experience is inseparable from such ideas and if the concepts of objective world, experience, and experiential route can be grasped only simultaneously. What matters for us here is the account of how facts about the more immediately available part of the structure can support, without any quasi-reduction, conclusions about the E-truths of this system of H.E., the remainder of the structure. For we who nonreflectively operate the spatial scheme of H.E., it is natural to raise this question as a problem about how, if our experience (*sic*) were different, we would infer to conclusions about the particular spatial structure of our world, our location in it, and what it is like at various places:

---

[5] It may be objected that this story is too thin to allow the legitimate application of the concept of a hallucination, and so derivatively the concept of an objective world. One source for such a claim would be the view that acquisition and application of the idea of a hallucination goes in step with the acquisition of *a posteriori* knowledge about what can disturb perception of the world. In reply to this claim I would make two points.

(a) The example in the footnote of Chapter I, p. 13, can easily be altered to one in which the connection between the world and the perceiver's experience is probabilistic, hallucinations resulting on certain occasions. If such examples are genuine possibilities, the objector's general claim is not true.

(b) More important, we could easily add to our story some perceptible quality a certain time after the perception of which the experiencer would hallucinate temporarily. This would not damage the important point of the story, viz. the role of the empirical theory of regularity.

but it is not essential that the question be so formulated.

As against all this, it may be said that the empirical theory of regularity plays such a large role in distinguishing the preplace at which the experiencer is located only because we have deprived him of two resources that are usually available to us when establishing our location, viz. (a) our ability to move ourselves and (b) our ability to discover traces of earlier qualities at a preplace. Thus at time t_3 the experiencer might intentionally move himself towards preplace 2, or again at t_4 he may notice traces of quality K.

Both these suggestions are completely mistaken if they are meant to show that the experiencer would not then need to rely on an empirical theory of regularity. Anything the experiencer intentionally does or tries to do to move himself from one preplace to another needs to be independently certified as doing just that, and so the experiencer must have some empirically confirmed theory that will ratify such actions as indeed producing change of preplace; the empirical theory of change at the preplaces is needed to do this. It is true that when an action has been discovered by the experiencer to move him, his doing so in some circumstances may allow him to draw distinctions he would not otherwise be able to make in these circumstances (a good example is the move from 1 to 2 just before t_0): but it does not provide a wholly independent source of evidence. This is even more obvious in the case of traces: to check that one feature is a trace of another, observation is useless unless one has the premise that one has remained at the same preplace. These two suggestions just illustrate the compelling general claim that no qualitative feature of experience can by itself logically ensure any truth about the spatial provenance of that experience, or about the spatial relation of its source to the sources of other experiences. This truth is just one of the irreducibility principles of Chapter I, section 1 in another guise.[6]

[6] In any case an ability to move oneself could not be essential to mastery of the spatial scheme, for there could be creatures with mastery of it who could not move themselves at all. Agreed, they must be able to perform some kinds of action if any attitudes are to be attributed to them at all; but these actions could be qualitative changes of the exterior of their bodies. The intelligent use of complex qualitative changes could make it unreasonable not to attribute beliefs about places to such creatures. (A detailed example could be given, but it would be tedious for it would show little more than has already been claimed.)

A second essential component of our experiencer's ability to draw the required distinctions is his memory of his experiences, not only of which experiences he has had earlier, but also of their *order*: it is plain that possession of a theory of the world which he knows to be true and without exceptions would not help him at all in establishing truths about his location if all he could remember was his experience of the previous time interval, or if he remembered all his experiences, but not their temporal ordering. There is a sense in which it is quite impossible for the spatio-temporal scheme of holistic explanation to be explanatory of only one's present experiences, and there is a sense in which memory must be cumulative in a stronger sense than is given by mere accumulation of beliefs and memory images of one's past. (This is a consequence of the point that the intertemporal constraint on the application of the E-concepts in the spatio-temporal scheme of holistic explanation concerns a system of spatially related places, where the relations can be investigated empirically by the experiencer only by means of his temporally successive observations.) There are a number of connected conclusions that can be drawn from this observation,[7] but the temptation is going to be resisted here in order

---

[7] For instance it suggests that a certain position that combines scepticism about the past existence of an objective world with a lack of scepticism about its present existence is incoherent. For in virtue of the latter half of the position, a distinction will be drawn between those present experiences that are of the objective world and those that are not. But there is no basis for drawing such a distinction, nor for expecting any particular consequences from it, unless one's apparent memories are taken seriously as evidence of a path followed in the past.

A second consequence is this. On pp. 227–9 of *Kant's Analytic*, Jonathan Bennett notes that we often use regularities about the objective world in settling the objective order of two remembered events: for the time of an event is not a 'perceptible feature of it'. This method of settling the order of course holds generally for anything that is not such a perceptible feature, and not only temporal order: thus I may settle the question of whether a speech I remember hearing was being given in Rome or London from my memory of the temperature in the vicinity; or again can decide that the substance I was examining yesterday was radioactive when I remember that I took it from a container marked in a certain way. But it is of great importance that this resource is available only after a well-confirmed theory of the objective order of events of the kind in question. We may be able to accommodate considerably more disconnected perceptions when it is so established than before, but the application of the scheme in the first place must rest on more direct memory of temporal order, of the kind involved when one remembers hearing a tune, the kind that Bennett (ibid., p. 228) construes in terms of a sequence of overlapping specious presents.

not to delay for too long a return to the structure of the main argument.

Why have I persisted in speaking of prespace and preplaces rather than space and places? Consider the case in which the sensory qualities F, G, . . . , L are perceptible by a sense modality that is not intrinsically spatial, say sounds or smells. In the diagram on p. 182 above I drew the four preplaces in the configuration of a square: but it seems clear that in this case, the fact that the preplaces are so arranged is something that has no consequences in the experience of a being whose sensory experiences are not spatial. All that he has access to in experience, and makes use of in his construction of a theory of his world, is an adjacency relation between preplaces, a relation that he works out to hold between 1 and 2, 2 and 3, 3 and 4, 4 and 1, and which he discovers to be symmetrical. (Of course a notationally different theory agreeing with all the facts of such a being's experience would be one which had infinitely many preplaces strung, so to speak, along one dimension, with infinite repetition. This would be analogous to the way in which finite genuinely spatial three-dimensional universes may be described instead as infinite.) If our experiencer were really operating with a spatial scheme, there must be some determinate answer, calculable from what is available to the experiencer, to the question of the shape in which the four distinct places are arranged. (It would be calculated in the same sense that the shape of Australia was worked out before space travel.) One way of showing vividly that no such answer can be given is this. We might actually set up an apparatus in which some newly born creature was deprived of all sensory capacities other than non-spatial ones, and was allowed to move between just four places with a history as in our diagram. This creature might be allowed the power of movement in the two directions around the cycle of the four places 1–4; though of course we would have to block off those nerves that would give indications that the creature was accelerating in one direction (in our space) rather than another. Now the point that nothing in the creature's experience possibly justifies saying that 1–4 are arranged in a square rather than some other configuration is reflected in this fact: in our set-up for this creature, it does not matter under the conditions we have imposed whether the places in our space that are his 1–4 are in the form of a square, a diamond, or any other four-sided figure. The particular spatial configuration employed has no effect on his course of experience. This way of making the point vivid should also make it plain that there need be no suggestion in the distinction that lies behind this talk of preplaces that there could be a prespace that was not in fact part of a real space: the point is rather one concerned with the degree of sophistication of the concepts of the objective used by the experiencer.

A charge might be made that the abilities that can be manifested in the prespatial world constitute no more than various sensori-motor skills: just as Piaget plausibly said that the abilities of a child of a few months manifest themselves in, but do not display a grasp of concepts of, space,[8] so a similar claim might be made about the being in our example and concepts of prespace. Now of course the ability to move oneself, considered on its own, is always just a sensori-motor skill: the important question is whether we can conceive of actions carried out in the prespatial world to which it is no less arbitrary to deny the title of manifestations of beliefs about prespace, than it is to deny the title of manifestations of beliefs about space to comparable spatial examples. Here are three examples of actions that may be performed in the prespatial world that appear to have that status, examples that could be both expanded and multiplied. First, we can imagine different responses by some being exposed to the course of experience in our example according to whether a type of sequence of experiences indicates change of preplace by the experiencer or change at a given preplace in the circumstances in which it occurs. For instance, when there is change of preplace the being may also go in a different direction if he needs to in order to obtain food, which we might suppose always to be given in the same preplace. Second, we may have evidence of an intelligent activity of circumnavigating obstacles to a desired destination in prespace. Third, some desired effects, if, say, they come about after exposure to three of the qualities F, G, . . . , L in a certain order, may require the experiencer to visit certain

[8] *The Child's Construction of Reality*, transl. M. Cook (London: Routledge and Kegan Paul, 1955), Chapter II, section 1.

preplaces at certain times to gain exposure to those qualities; again it will in sophisticated cases be hard not to see his activities as manifestations of the employment of prespatial concepts. If, in a more complex prespatial world, we admit more preplaces and allow other beings and allow them to produce some perceptible qualities themselves, we can even allow the beings with experience of only a prespatial world to express and communicate their prespatial judgements in language.

I have concentrated on the prespatial example in setting up this half of the comparison with the action explanation case, partly for its novelty and intrinsic interest, and partly for the reason that it abstracts from complications irrelevant to our present purpose that arise when the senses involved are intrinsically spatial. Nevertheless, it ought to be clear that if we had chosen a genuinely spatial and not a prespatial example, the theory of regularity would still have played the same major role in establishing a theory of the objective world without use of a quasi-reduction: the points really important to the general comparison needed for the account of holistic explanation being proposed are common to the prespatial and the spatial cases. Given the distinction between the prespatial and the spatial worlds, it is clear too that there is a need for a philosophical investigation to be carried out upon another occasion into the precise way in which the spatiality of an experiencer's world relates to the spatiality of his senses: we would want to know how the spatial features of his world have their seeds in, grow from, spatial features intrinsic to the deliverances of the senses he has.

We can have empirical evidence that a dog believes of a particular place that its bone is buried *there*, rather than (say) under the pile of leaves: the evidence would consist in such facts as that if we move the pile of leaves, the dog still searches where the leaves were, and not at the new location of the pile. Does this mean that we have to say that the dog makes inferences to the best explanation of his experiences in accordance with the *a priori* principles and the intertemporal constraints? Surely we should not want to attribute grasp of even the concept of experience to the dog at all!

The reply to this objection is analogous to that in Chapter I to the objection that someone can knowledgeably apply the concepts of belief, desire, and intention without ever having contemplated the *a priori* principles and intertemporal constraints. Provided that the mechanism productive of noninferential belief that it's ϕ at a certain place operates in such a way as to produce the same beliefs that would be produced if the principles were consciously applied, nothing here contradicts our account. In the case of the dog in particular, we can see that the dog, in its journey to the place where it believes the bone to be, is causally influenced by exactly what it would be influenced by if it were applying the E-concepts in the way we have described.

It is unnecessary to set out a case corresponding in detail to the four preplace or more sophisticated examples, in order to see that precisely analogous considerations to those raised several pages ago apply to the attribution of beliefs and desires to a person and to the interpretation of his utterances. In so far as both a course of experience and a sequence of behaviour are explained in their respective schemes of H.E. by the application of a pair of E-concepts, any given course of experience or sequence of behaviour may *prima facie* be explained in a number of different ways; in particular, one may always hang on to the supposition that the agent has a given attitude, or the experiencer a given location, if one makes enough compensating adjustments elsewhere. Why do we pick one explanation rather than another? If our basic claim about the parallelism between the action and the perceptual cases is correct, to ask this is to ask the question: what for the action case is the analogue of the theory of regularity?

It cannot just be rationality, however broadly construed: for that we saw to be the intertemporal constraint on the application of the E-concepts of the action scheme, and I argued that the spatial analogue of that was continuity of motion. The analogue of the theory of regularity of properties at places has in the action case to be a theory of regularity of such nonrational factors as the constancy and change of underived desires (desires that are not derivative from other desires) over time, and the connection of sensory stimuli physically characterized with the formation of beliefs.[9] There is a further certain rough symmetry here. In the perceptual case, the supposition of

[9] Compare the discussion in Chapter I, section 4, above of an agent's belief that a given object is red.

continuity of motion and a statement of location of a perceiver at a given time have no consequences for which sequences of experiences are empirically possible for the perceiver until we adjoin a statement of the theory of regularity – what it's like at the places over time. Similarly for action; the supposition of rationality and what is believed at a given time have no particular consequences for empirically possible sequences of actions until we adjoin a theory of the agent's underived desires over time, and have also an account of such matters as the connection of his beliefs with sensory stimuli.[10]

Once we have distinguished the empirical theory of regularity from the intertemporal constraints, the fact that in the action case there are many persons while there is only one public, common space becomes an important difference between the two schemes. For a given range of perceptible properties, the relevant empirical theory of regularity is the same for all perceivers able to perceive that range: for the regularities concern the objective properties of places in space. It is not similarly true that for a given range of actions that may be performed, the relevant empirical theory of regularity is the same for all agents with that range of abilities: for the regularities concern stimuli, psychological states, and changes of psychological states. The intertemporal rationality constraint may be the same for all rational agents, but we have distinguished that from the empirical theory of regularity. The significance of the existence of many persons, then, is that for persons of a given species or some other chosen kind, one may be able to reason inductively from the empirical theory of regularity for one member of the kind to the correct theory of regularity for another member. Similarly one can build up a theory of empirical regularity for a typical member of a kind from the behaviour of many different particular members of the kind.

There are some fascinating issues which I leave here in order to state in verbally parallel fashion for the action and interpretation cases the earlier account in this section of what

---

[10] There is also of course an asymmetry: a regularity theory in the perceptual case provides truths of the form 'it's ϕ at place p', and in the action case is concerned partly with underived desires. But in the tightest way of stating the parallel in Chapter I, 'it's ϕ at place p' was compared with *belief*. The general claim, then, can only be that a theory of regularity governing *some* E-concepts is needed.

allows us to apply the E-concepts in the spatial case. The statement is as follows. Any sequence of behaviour whatever is such that we can assign a (possibly changing) pattern of beliefs, desires, and sentence senses that would rationally explain it; but many of these sequences provide in themselves no basis for the distinctions we can draw between propositional attitudes changing and different attitudes already possessed becoming operative, or indeed, in some cases, sentence sense changing. Such distinctions can only be drawn with the help of empirical hypotheses about the stability of desires and, for instance, beliefs about what is evidence for what; again, it is a regularity not in the facts explained, but in truths stated using the E-concepts of the scheme, that is in question. (So reductionists were right to advert to regularities, but mislocated the vocabulary in which they need to be stated.) Corresponding to the observations we made about memory, we have the point that, unless we have inductive evidence from the behaviour of other creatures of the same kind, we cannot apply the scheme to a creature without some considerable knowledge of his past behaviour: one cannot set out using the scheme knowledgeably *ab initio*.

It may be felt that there is an asymmetry between the action and the spatial schemes in respect of the role of time in each of them. This is not a question of whether each scheme is concerned with explaining change over time: for in both cases we are concerned to provide a theory of the application of the E-concepts over time in a way that explains temporally extended courses of action or perception. But it might be said that there is a difference if we consider the applications of the E-concepts of each scheme to an object at a given time. The beliefs and desires a person has at a given time, in the logical structure of the sentences specifying their content, exhibit the relations of content which are subject to the intertemporal constraints and, which make the action scheme holistic in our sense. But the features displayed at a place at a time do not in the corresponding way capture the holistic features of the spatial scheme: for those features involve the concept of a (really) possible continuous path, and this imposes constraints only when we have specified how the E-concepts apply at other times.

I protest that this is not a fair comparison given the analogy that is being proposed. The analogue in the spatial scheme of the possession of a belief by an agent in the action scheme is not just the display of a quality, but the instantiation of a property at a given place. But then the parallelism is restored, because just as it is essential to a belief that it have the relations of content it does to other attitudes, equally it is essential to a given place that it have the spatial relations it does to other places. (The same holds for preplaces and prespatial relations.) When the analogy is stated properly, at least three specific points of parallelism emerge even when we so restrict attention to a given time t. (a) The features at places other than the one at which the experiencer is located at t are not actually explanatory (in the required way) of experiences at t just as an agent's nonoperative beliefs and desires at t are not explanatory of his behaviour at t, but (b) these nonoperative states are in both cases potentially explanatory of experience or action by the *a priori* principles of the scheme if things had been different (his spatial location or the circumstances relevant to action), and (c) in both cases this potential relevance is subject both to the qualification that the hypothetically changed location or circumstances do not affect the application of the E-concepts of the scheme of explanation, and to the intertemporal restrictions.

There is indeed a different difference relating to time in the two schemes. Suppose that over a lengthy period a man acts in accordance with the beliefs and desires which we attribute to him; and then unexpectedly ϕ's intentionally for some ϕ which the beliefs and desires we have so far attributed to him do not rationalize. Say he acts this unexpected way at t_0. Now in the action case we have two quite distinct kinds of resource for accounting for his ϕ-ing intentionally: either we can say that his beliefs themselves have changed, or we may say that they have not, but that he always had a belief that t_0 or some interval surrounding it is different in some respects from earlier times (and similarly for desires). There can of course be good empirical grounds for choosing an explanation of one of these kinds over one of the other kind: the point at present is just that both are available in principle, and there seems to be nothing quite analogous to this in the spatial case. The question is whether this difference is a sign of some new structural feature of the action case, additional to the differences already noted between it and the spatial case, that destroys any arguments presupposing a parallelism. It seems it is not such an additional feature since its source is just that beliefs and desires have contents, are specified by 'that . . .' clauses: for this immediately allows the possibility of a belief that is about a particular time or interval. No further source is needed to account for the difference.

I have repeatedly asserted that there is no quasi-reduction of the spatial scheme of holistic explanation. But there is in fact a suggestion by Poincaré made first in *Science and Hypothesis* and expanded later in *The Value of Science* that might be regarded as an important part of a quasi-reduction of the spatial scheme.[11] Poincaré said that one could distinguish a change of position of an object (other than oneself, and relative to oneself) from a change of state of some external object, thus: in the case of a change of position, by making certain bodily movements, such as turning the head, one can 'correct' for the change and restore one's original perceptual state, while in the case of a change of state externally one cannot thus restore the original perceptual state.

Poincaré's suggestion, if it could be worked up in the way he evidently hoped, would at most be part of a quasi-reduction rather than a full reduction, because to apply it one evidently needs to know that one's experiences are of an objective world, and not hallucinatory states: so clause (i) of the definition of a quasi-reduction is met. Viewing the suggestion as part of a quasi-reduction is charitable to it in another respect too. It answers some of Piaget's objections[12] to Poincaré's account to note that viewed as part of a quasi-reduction, the person to whom the suggestion is supposed to be of some help will indeed have the general idea of an external universe as composed of 'substantial and permanent' objects – what, in parallel with other quasi-reductions, he will not have is knowledge of the particular disposition of objects and changes of position and state that there actually are in the world.

The criterion Poincaré gives is of course clearly incorrect: the test given for change of position is neither sufficient nor neces-

[11] *Science and Hypothesis* (New York: Scott, 1905), Chapter IV, and *The Value of Science* (New York: Dover, 1958), Chapter III.
[12] *The Child's Construction of Reality*, pp. 102–13.

sary. It is not sufficient since a bodily movement may allow
one to perceive an object qualitatively similar to that which
one was perceiving before it changed: and it is not necessary
since a moving object may also change. These observations are
in themselves banal: what is of interest is rather their status in
the spatial scheme of holistic explanation. For here we see that
the reason a proposed quasi-reduction is not adequate is that
with our full mastery of the scheme, we can see how an application of the concept Q of the quasi-reduction can fail to be
evidence of a pattern of application of the E-concepts of the
scheme, and this on the basis of our understanding of the ways
in which the application of the E-concepts could combine, all
the time in accordance with the *a priori* principles of the
scheme, to produce the 'misleading' application of the concept
Q. (The analogue of this example in the propositional attitude
scheme would be a case in which an apparently sincere assertion
could be seen not to be so when a detailed assignment of
beliefs, desires, and sentence senses is established.)

Poincaré's suggestion cannot be general for another reason.
One cannot perceive by the sense of touch objects that are not
in contact with any part of one's body. Yet the congenitally
blind, whose space is a purely haptic one, are able to distinguish
inferentially in at least some cases between change of position
and change of state of an object at some distance from them:
therefore Poincaré's method cannot be the only basis for
drawing the distinction. It is also of interest that the examples
Poincaré actually gives all concern the changes of position or
state of an object in the visual field throughout the change.

Many questions arise once the general parallelism between
the action and spatial cases suggested here is granted. One first
thought, for instance, concerns uniqueness and indeterminacy.
There seems to be no plausibility in the idea that there is any
more than ordinary inductive uncertainty over the uniqueness
of the everyday assignment of ordinary objects and features to
places. If that is so, there is no necessary connection between
the holistic nature of a system of explanation and multiplicity
of complete sets of E-truths that explain the B-facts of the system.
But the thought I want to develop here starts rather from the
point that in our simple prespatial example we have a relatively
clear conception of how we can come to apply the E-concepts

without possessing a quasi-reduction for the system. This possibility raises questions about Davidson's radical interpretation procedure.

2. RADICAL INTERPRETATION

Davidson's radical interpretation procedure rests in part upon the attitude of holding a sentence true, which is 'one special kind of belief, the belief that a sentence is true';[13] and it is said that this attitude can in effect play the crucial role of a concept Q in a quasi-reduction because

We can know that a speaker holds a sentence to be true without knowing what he means by it or what belief it expresses for him.[14]

Now the concept of holding a sentence true has an analogue we should consider in the spatial case, that of being ϕ-located: a person is ϕ-located at a time iff he is at that time located somewhere where it is then ϕ. It is equally the case that a man can know that he is ϕ-located without knowing where he is or which place it is that is ϕ, as for instance on waking after having been transported during sleep and set down on the shore at Ithaca. In the case of ϕ-location, this is possible because the concept has been defined by an existentially quantified condition, and in general one can know that something meets a condition without knowing of any particular object that it does. Does a similar explanation apply to the corresponding possibility for holding-true?

Strictly we should note that Davidson has never defined holding-true by this kind of existential quantification: he has always said that to hold a sentence s true is to have a certain belief, the belief that s is true. Nevertheless I shall argue that the explanation of the possibility by existential quantification that we just suggested for the case of ϕ-location, is correct in the case of holding-true also. First, note that the Davidsonian definition is not quite what we need as evidence in radical interpretation: if I do not speak Serbo-Croat, the fact that, perhaps on the basis of testimony, I believe certain sentences of Serbo-Croat to be true is not relevant in the ascription to me of ground level, nonsemantical beliefs. The same applies to

---

[13] 'Belief and the Basis of Meaning', p. 316.
[14] 'Thought and Talk', p. 14; see also 'Radical Interpretation'.

sentences of the language of my own speech community that contain expressions that I do not understand. My belief that s is true is evidence that I have the belief that s expresses only in cases in which for some p, s in a fragment of a language I understand says that p. So in the only cases that are relevant to belief ascription, x's holding s true can be defined as: for some p, s in a language x fully understands says that p, and x believes that p. And this definition has a similar existentially quantified form to that of 'ϕ-location'.

This may seem an unfair manœuvre against Davidson. Why should he not say that holding a sentence true as he defines it is always *evidence* that a person believes what is said by the sentence, even if the evidence can be overriden? But to say this would be to overlook the role of holding-true in his radical interpretation procedure: this procedure requires that if x holds-true s and the procedure delivers the answer that s has the truth condition that p, then x believes that p. As Davidson says, 'If we know he holds the sentence true *and* we know how to interpret it, then we can make a correct attribution of belief.'[15] Were Davidson to abandon this principle, then he could not really regard the theory of 'Belief and the Basis of Meaning' as solving the problem it set out to answer. If holding-true is going to conform to this principle, then we must not allow that a person can hold true sentences that he does not understand.

There is a subtle and a less subtle response to this argument. The less subtle one is to say that the principle should be qualified by addition of 'and if there is no strong evidence independent of the interpretation procedure that x does not believe that p' to its antecedent. This is a weak reply since if there can be evidence independent of the radical interpretation procedure about detailed beliefs, why did we need the radical interpretation procedure in the first place? The more subtle reply is to use a Davidsonian tactic the second time around, and say that one can know that someone does not have the belief expressed by a sentence he believes true without knowing which belief it does express. This is true: but it is important that this is now a possibility claim that *is* true because of its

---

[15] 'Thought and Talk', p. 14. Cp. also 'Belief and the Basis of Meaning', p. 313: 'Given the interpretations, we could read off beliefs from the evidential base . . .'.

(negative) existential character. The arguments of the text below can be generalized to apply to it.

There is yet another complication to be discussed before we reach the main argument. Even when sentence s is a sentence of x's language, it may be that x holds true s and yet there is no p such that x believes that p and s in x's language says that p. For if, for instance, s contains a vacuous name, then s does not say anything at all. We cannot say that someone who sincerely asserts 'Vulcan is smaller than Mercury' believes that Vulcan is smaller than Mercury: since 'Vulcan' does not denote, we do not attribute any belief to the asserter in saying that at all. There may be associated descriptive beliefs, but these are not what the sentence expresses. Hence the definition of 'holds true' in terms of existential quantification is not strictly correct. We might try to repair the definition by requiring that only sentences which say something are to be counted as part of a person's language: but it is clear that on this notion of language, one must already have done a considerable amount of radical interpretation before one can determine which sentences are and which are not in someone's language.

The important point for us is that such cases do not throw doubt on the condition that if someone holds true a sentence s, then for any p, if s says that p then x believes that p. (This needs further qualification if s is ambiguous.) This condition is still a quantification of a predicate containing 'x believes that p', where 'p' is a variable associated with a range of sentences that express detailed beliefs. The quantification is now a universal quantification, but that does not matter for the argument to be given below. I will continue to give the argument for the naïve existential quantifier form of definition but the arguments to be given will work for any quantification of a predicate that is or contains 'believes'.

Now it seems clear that one is able to know one is ϕ-located without knowing where one is or where it is that is ϕ, only because one's experiences are of a kind previously obtained as experiences of an objective world, and to know that one was having such experiences one would need to have been operating in the past with some theory, however rudimentary, of one's path in an objective spatial world, with the ability to make particular applications of the E-concepts: one would need to have been able in the past to know where one was located and what it was like at that particular place. By this, I do not mean merely that one must in the past have had a general conceptual ability that has no specific connection with the present judgement 'I am now ϕ-located': on the contrary, I mean that one must in the past (or must now see that one was in the past in a position to) have judged that one was at a particular (a certain) place, and that place was then ϕ, and that one's present experience is of a kind (such as Odysseus' experience of the seashore) that one had when one knew oneself to be ϕ-located on more direct grounds such as we have already discussed.[16] Being an inductive inference, this step is naturally not *prima facie* invulnerable to various sceptical challenges: the important point for us at present is that in the relevant respects it exactly parallels the following kind of case involving propositional attitudes and holding-true. Let us consider circumstances in which we know a man to hold a sentence true, on the basis of honest assertion, but do not know what belief of his it expresses. We may know the sentence is held true because we know whenever he speaks in that straightforward tone of voice, he is speaking honestly, and we know, say, he speaks more quickly when trying to deceive, in a different tone when ironic, and so on; it just happens that on this occasion our speaker is using arcane vocabulary to his scientific colleagues. It seems clear in this case that our justification for our belief that the scientific sentence is held true must make reference to our earlier success in attributing beliefs on the supposition that such utterances are honest, just as Odysseus' justification for his belief that he is ϕ-located must make reference to earlier analogous successes. (In both cases of course it is not required that one remember which were the occasions on which such hypotheses proved successful: one needs only to know that there were such successes.)[17]

[16] By using 'judged' in this sentence I do not mean to imply that when one has the kind of inductive evidence here in question that one is ϕ-located, one must earlier have had experiences sufficient to meet sceptical challenges about whether one was experiencing an objective world at all. It is sufficient for the present point that one earlier 'worked the system' in the sense that one knew what a nonsceptical operator would have been prepared to assert about his location and the objective world, given such experiences.

[17] Another example to which an argument of the same general form can be applied is given by Wittgenstein: 'But how does the observer distinguish . . . between players' mistakes and correct play? – There are characteristic signs of it

If this is correct, we may say that an account, if one could be given, of how to determine a specific system of features, objects, and places in which the experiencer traces a path taking the notion of ϕ-location as the putative concept with the role of Q, would not provide a quasi-reduction of the spatial system of holistic explanation. For in the cases so far considered at least, while it is true that one may know one is ϕ-located without knowing where one is located and which place it is that is ϕ, one can know this only if one has earlier been able to make judgements involving specific applications to particular objects of the E-concepts of the system of holistic explanation in question. But it was precisely such applications of the E-concepts of the system that the quasi-reduction was meant to deliver rather than presuppose.

It is important to avoid a possible confusion about the parallel just given. One expression of the starting-point of the confusion would be this:

> In the parallel just given, the analogues of nonveridical experiences are deceptive utterances (or more strictly, utterances that are sayings of things the utterer does not believe). But in the parallel developed at the start of this section, deceptive utterances or actions would not be the analogues of nonveridical experiences: for plainly deceptive utterances, just like nondeceptive ones, are explained in terms of the agent's beliefs, desires, and intentions: these are not cases where the application of the scheme lapses, as it does in the case of involuntary bodily movements, spasms, and so forth. Since different parallels are evidently in question, there is no transfer from the parallel developed earlier to the present issues about holding-true.

All these remarks are acceptable except the final sentence. It is indeed the case that in terms of the parallel given at the start of this section, the analogue of the concept 'x is ϕ-located at t' would in the belief and desire version be:

---

in the players' behaviour. Think of the behaviour characteristic of correcting a slip of the tongue. It would be possible to recognize that someone was doing so even without knowing his language.' *Philosophical Investigations*, section 54 (Oxford: Blackwell, 2nd edition, 1958).

$\exists p\ \exists\psi(x$ believes at t that if he ψ's at the time he believes t to be then p, and desires that p and can and believes he can ψ);
in the version using intention, which we saw a long way back to be needed strictly speaking, the corresponding concept would be:
$\exists\psi(x$ intends at t to ψ at the time he believes t to be).
But to conclude to an objection from the truth that in the more recent parallel we were comparing ϕ-location with a more limited concept, that relates to only part of the holistic scheme of action-explanation, viz. holding-true, would be to have misunderstood much of the rest of the argument. For one of the features of the distinctive concepts of a scheme of holistic explanation is that such concepts cannot be properly applied unless they conform to the rationality constraints upon the intertemporal applications of the E-concepts of the scheme. There are two distinctions in play in the objection: (1) the distinction between deceptive and honest utterances, and (2) the distinction between events that are intentional and those that are not. The objector is in effect suggesting that we can apply distinction (1) without taking into account the claims made earlier in this chapter about distinction (2). But each half of the distinction (1) presupposes the utterance is intentional under some description; and the application of distinction (2) I have suggested requires the assignment of detailed beliefs and desires. But this will settle which utterances are deceptive and which are honest. There is not the independence of (1) and (2) that the objector claims. I will argue in more detail in a few pages that an instance of holding-true can be certified as such ultimately only by reference to a theory of the agent's beliefs, desires, and sentence senses that is adequately rationally explanatory of his actions and has the holding-true in question as a consequence.

The case of ϕ-location shows that we need to distinguish at least two different ways in which the application of a concept may be said to 'assume' things about the application of other concepts. I cannot emphasize this distinction too strongly. In 'On the Very Idea of a Conceptual Scheme', Davidson writes that in radical interpretation we need 'a theory which rests on evidence that assumes neither [attitudes nor interpretation]' (p. 18). There are two ways 'assume' might be taken here.

(1) It might mean that there is no entailment from an evidence-specifying sentence using the concept of holding-true to sentences saying what (in general, nonsemantical) belief the sentence held true expresses, nor is there any entailment about what the sentence means. Evidence-sentences employing 'holds true' do indeed make no such assumption, and this is so just because of the existential nature of its definition. But this is quite compatible with its making assumptions in a second sense (2), according to which evidence-specifying sentences make assumptions about the application of other concepts only when the evidence-sentence itself cannot be established except in the context of a theory attributing detailed beliefs, meanings, and intentions to the person said to hold the sentence true. Now the difficulty facing the radical interpreter in the way Davidson states the problem is met only if no assumptions in sense (2) are made. One role of the spatial analogy is to show that the concept of ϕ-location makes no corresponding assumptions in sense (1): that is, a sentence to the effect that x is ϕ-located at t does not for any particular place p entail that it is ϕ at p at t. Nevertheless we have seen that it is plausible that such a sentence about ϕ-location cannot be established without invoking a theory of routes through a spatial world, albeit possibly of a rudimentary kind, which prevents the concept from being free of assumptions with respect to place in sense (2).[18]

Though I have adverted so far to only one kind of case in arguing for the inability of holding-true to function as the concept Q of a quasi-reduction, the arguments for the impossibility of its doing so are entirely general: it is unnecessary to argue riskily from a few particular examples. The more general argument may be initially stated thus.

[18] Someone might maintain a position analogous to Davidson's on radical interpretation and holding-true generally: the claims would be that one can know that someone is acting intentionally under some description without knowing which particular description it is, and that this fact gives a special role to the notion of acting intentionally under some description in attributing to an agent a pattern of beliefs and desires. (A full statement of the position would have to come up with something playing a role analogous to the role of the Principle of Charity in Davidson's procedure.) It will not come as a surprise by this stage that I would maintain that the concept of acting intentionally under some description fails to make assumptions about the intentions of the agent in sense (1), but not in sense (2); the arguments given about holding-true and the spatial parallel may be reproduced equally for the notion of acting intentionally under some description.

The central kind, though not the only kind, of evidence for the presence of the attitude of holding-true is honest assertion. We can infer from the evidence of utterances that an assertion is honest, as Davidson himself notes, only if we 'know much about [the speaker's] desires and beliefs':[19] moreover, it is not just knowledge of his desirings-true and believings-true that we need. We need knowledge of such finely discriminated beliefs and desires as the desire that one's interlocutor be not mis-informed, the absence of any belief that he is counter-suggestible, and so forth; and even the more realistic attribution of a general disposition to honesty requires a skeletal knowledge of the subject's beliefs and desires. These will be yielded only by the application of a system of holistic explanation to the speaker's actions, including his utterances. It is a point Davidson has made time and again against reductive construals of Grice's programme that finely discriminated propositional attitudes cannot be attributed to a language-using creature in advance of systematic interpretation of his utterances; and the point operates here to show that the attitude of holding-true cannot play the role of a central concept Q in a quasi-reduction of this scheme of holistic explanation.[20]

[19] 'Thought and Talk', p. 14.
[20] It may be said that there is an asymmetry that has been overlooked here between

(a) the judgements Odysseus reaches if in his new circumstances he does not make inductive inferences from previous experience kinds, but instead establishes anew a theory of the region he is now in and concludes that his first experience in it was indeed veridical, and

(b) the analogous judgements we make about a man's attitudes when producing from scratch a theory that explains his actions.

For in (b) it may be said that the judgements we reach say what the agent believes and desires; whereas it cannot be said in case (a) that Odysseus need know where he is located, in that he need not know whether he is on the Aegean as opposed to the Mediterranean shore, etc. So a symmetry in terms of 'knowing where' will not hold. And it would be too weak to maintain that in case (a) Odysseus obtains judgements expressible in the form 'I am at p' where 'p' is replaced by a proper name of a place. (By introducing new proper names, he can do that before establishing the theory: he will certainly be connected with each place in a way that allows him properly to introduce a name of that very place, and express beliefs of it in using that name.) What then is the parallel?

We said earlier that spatial relations between places play a role in the spatial system of holistic explanation parallel to that played by relations between contents of beliefs and desires in the action case. It is here that the parallel lies in this case too. In case (a), Odysseus must not merely make judgements about particular places; he must also have an at least skeletal theory of the spatial relations between

3. A FULLER ARGUMENT

The above argument may seem hasty and incomplete. It can be filled out by considering the following exhaustive and exclusive classification of cases into one of which must fall any quasi-reduction for the propositional attitude scheme that takes as its concept Q the notion of holding-true.

(1) It may be held that we can identify the incidence of holding-true without any use of a theory of the agent's beliefs and desires at all. It would fly in the face of the facts to attribute such an implausible view to Davidson, who in at least two places asserts that some such knowledge of beliefs and desires is needed.[21] Indeed, to deny that would be in some respect to deny the holism of the mental, since holding-true is tied to belief, the ascription of which is tied to constraints involving desires.

(2) A second position would be that while we need some knowledge of beliefs and desires in order to determine what is held true, the attitudes needed are not those for the ascription of which we need the very interpretation the quasi-reduction involving holding-true was meant to deliver. It is perhaps such a position Davidson has in mind when he wrote that 'we can tell when a speaker holds a sentence to be true without knowing . . . what *detailed* intentions do or might prompt him to utter it.'[22] (My emphasis.) It would be an error to think that the example given earlier of a man uttering an arcane scientific sentence, where it could be inductively identified that he held it true, would necessarily be an example in conformity with this second position. For in that example it may remain that, in the area in which a certain style of assertion was identified as evidence of sincere expression of belief, there were attitudes which had to be present for an utterance to be a sign of holding-true, but which yet could have their presence certified only by

---

them, in the way that in (b) we need at least an outline of the contents of (some of) the agent's beliefs and desires. It is not to be denied, however, that there are some strict standards that one can apply in connection with the phrase 'knowing where' that do not have analogues for 'knowing what' (in the case of attitudes), and for which different judgements for (a) and (b) are in order. 'Knowing where' and 'knowing when' may be somewhat special within the class 'knowing who/what/where/which/when/why . . .'.

[21] 'Thought and Talk', p. 14 and 'On the Very Idea', p. 18.
[22] 'Belief and the Basis of Meaning', p. 313.

a theory of meaning for the subject's sentences within the non-arcane area.

A truth that is relevant to the assessment of this second position and which we need to consider carefully is this. There is no propositional attitude, however detailed or theoretical in content or subject-matter, that cannot enter an agent's operative reasons for producing a deceptive utterance. A mathematician may desire to see a certain theorem proved, and believe that if he lies to his colleague, the latter is likely to spend his time attempting to prove it (rather than at the beach), and if he succeeds he will thereby contribute to the first mathematician's goals. So even the most theoretical beliefs may be amongst an agent's operative reasons for an action. The reason we have to be careful in assessing this truth is this: the specific detailed belief or desire that operatively rationalizes the deceptive utterance, provides the agent's reason for uttering a sentence having a certain content he does not in fact believe. But of course the radical interpretation procedures never in themselves initially required the identification of the specific content of the utterance: they require a sorting of the utterances into those events e such that there is some p such that e is a saying that p and the utterer of e believes that p, and those events e that lack this property. So we must not just beg the question by assuming that the desires and beliefs we have to attribute in advance to identify the holdings-true must also be sufficient to rationalize the utterance under a description 'saying that p' for some detailed p.

Nevertheless, these considerations do raise a query that need not involve begging the question. The following principle P seems to have great plausibility:

Someone can know what it is for something to be F only if he knows what it is for a particular thing to be F.   (P)

(Here 'a particular' has narrower scope than 'only if'.) There is a question of how to regiment this principle, for its second clause is not of the form:

only if $\exists x$(he knows what it is for x to be F).

But this does not detract from the point that 'a particular' in this sentence makes an intelligible difference from the reading of the sentence one would obtain if 'something' were put in its place. (It is for us to expand our representations of logical form to meet this point, not for us to restrict what we are allowed to say. The principle seems to be equally plausible when 'something' is a substitutional quantifier (with 'thing' reconstrued appropriately).[23]

P is immune from objections based on the fact that we sometimes accept existential quantifications on the authority of others while not understanding ourselves the predicate that is existentially quantified. In such circumstances, if the sentence accepted is 'Something is F', and we do not know what it is for particular objects to be F, then there is no answer to the charge that we do not understand the sentence; what we learn in that case is merely that a certain sentence expresses a truth. We do not come to know the truth it expresses, and so cannot be said to know that something is F; nor, therefore, does the fact that in the imagined example we do not know what it is for something to be F, contradict the principle P.[24]

P appears to pose a serious threat to the position (2) on Davidson's radical interpretation procedure that we are

---

[23] The analogous principle for universal quantification is: someone can know what it is for everything to be F only if he knows what it is for a particular thing to be F. This also seems to be true. Its truth is of course required for the correctness of my earlier claim that we could employ the existential definition of holding-true without loss of generality.

[24] Note that P is in some respects stronger and in some respects weaker than this principle PS:

> To understand sentences of the form ⌜Something is F⌝ one has to understand sentences of the form ⌜a is F⌝, where a is a singular term. (PS)

P applies in what seems to be a conceptually possible case: that of a language containing existentially quantified sentences but no singular terms. (One generalization of PS to other languages entails there cannot be languages with existential quantification but no singular terms.) But P is also weaker than PS in that it does not of itself require understanding of any singular sentences, even when they are in the language, in order for there to be understanding of existentially quantified sentences.

Not being a principle about sentences, P is not vulnerable to the objection that the present arguments based upon it could be circumvented by teaching someone 'holds-true' as an unstructured predicate. It is the possibility of such a reply that blocks off the route of dealing with case (2) by a quick appeal to the principle suggested by Dummett (*Frege: Philosophy of Language*, pp. 236–9 and elsewhere) that understanding of a sentence involves a grasp of the most 'direct' way of verifying it, that is of the way that goes in step with the semantically relevant syntactic structure of the sentence; the most direct way in the case of an existentially quantified sentence $\exists x\, F(x)$ is by finding something within the range of the existential quantifier and verifying that it meets the condition $F(\quad)$.

currently considering. As we have seen, the statement that a given person x holds a sentence s true may be taken to be of the form 'Something is F': for, subject to the qualifications made earlier, it expands to 'For some p, s in x's language says that p and x believes that p'. The threat in the application of P to holding-true is one of circularity. If Davidson's radical interpretation procedure is the only account of what it is for someone who has a language to believe that p, for some detailed particular p, then we are apparently in the following position. In order to know what it is to hold something true, we have to know what it is to have particular beliefs (by principle P),[25] and to know what it is for someone with a language to have particular beliefs we have to know what it is for him to hold a sentence true (by the nature of the radical interpretation procedure). So we seem to have a circle.

This objection may seem wholly misconceived, for the reason that 'a quasi-reduction was meant to be a means to the *application* of concepts already possessed, and not to be part of an account of knowledge of *what it is* for something to fall under the concept. Principle P is thus just simply inapplicable to the case.'

When I wrote in clause (i) of the definition of a quasi-reduction (p. 179 above) that Q could not be possessed by someone with no grasp whatsoever of the scheme of holistic explanation in question, this was meant to rule out a quasi-reduction from having a reduction: it does not exclude the possibility that on a quasi-reductive view, grasp of what it is (say) to believe that p requires grasp of the quasi-reductive method. (Of course we commonly attribute beliefs to one another with no thought of the quasi-reductive method: once again this need not matter to such a theorist if it can be shown that the ascriptions justified by our normal procedures must coincide with those delivered by the quasi-reduction.) Now I assume that our present quasi-reductionist will indeed say that grasp of what it is to believe that p requires grasp of the quasi-reductive method, for he needs an answer to an objection that takes the form of a dilemma. The dilemma starts from a very plausible link between meaning and confirmation. If someone knows what it is for it to be the case that p, then he must (at the

---

[25] In this step it is being assumed that to know what it is for $p\&q$ to be the case, one has to know what it is for q to be the case.

very weakest) be in possession of a conception from which he can potentially reason – recognize on presentation certain forms of reasoning – to *possible evidence* that it is the case that p (no doubt under the supposition of various auxiliary hypotheses). Now the quasi-reductionist is faced with the dilemma that either he denies this, or the possible evidence that can be reasoned to may be used to *circumvent* the use of the method M. The natural way out of this dilemma is for the quasi-reductionist to say that what it is for an E-concept to apply to an object is grasped simultaneously with the quasi-reduction (Q,M) for the scheme.

It might be replied to the circularity objection from principle P, that these necessary conditions which do lead to a circularity if one supposes that the necessary condition has in some sense to be fulfilled *prior* to that for which it is necessary, may nevertheless all be fulfilled simultaneously. I shall first query the possibility of simultaneous determination in this particular case, and then raise another difficulty that is present for anyone who regards a quasi-reduction of the notion of belief as mandatory, regardless of whether such a person holds that the argument from principle P is to be avoided by simultaneous determination or by some other means.

'Simultaneous' is a metaphor, and presumably the objector intends it to advert to simultaneous equations, simultaneous inductive definitions not being in question. If we are going to have the simultaneous determination of a pair of concepts, holding-true and belief, we will need a pair of conditions governing them. One connecting condition is given by Davidson's radical interpretation procedure itself: this links holding-true with belief, since if person x holds true sentence s, and as a result of the procedure's application s is found in x's language to say that p, then x believes that p. But the only other connection between the two that we have is the one derived from principle P itself. Now that connection is one that holds between *any* existentially quantified predicate and (one conjunct of) the predicate quantified: there is nothing in the holding of this connection that is special to belief and holding-true. But in that case, we seem to have too little to determine simultaneously a pair of concepts: as distinctive of the concepts to be fixed, we have only the connection supplied by the radical interpretation procedure itself, and that will be insufficient to help someone who, we are supposing in this case, has in advance neither the ability to judge when someone holds some given sentence true, nor the ability to make detailed ascriptions of belief. So the charge of circularity seems to stand.[26]

A second problem can be raised even if the reply appealing to simultaneity can be made to stand up. There are cases in which we ascribe beliefs and in which the ultimate basis of attribution cannot be the Davidsonian radical interpretation procedure: the two most obvious are the case of the ascription of beliefs to a creature that does not have a language at all, and the ascription to someone who does have a language of beliefs that are not in fact expressible in his language as it then is.[27] (Particularly if his language is weak in devices for making indexical reference, a person may have many beliefs that he cannot express in his language as it then is, about colours, tastes, places, times, physical magnitudes, and so forth.) Since there are such cases, anyone who wishes to defend the view that a quasi-reduction involving holding-true is an indispensable method in ascribing beliefs to persons that do have a language, will have to say why one and the same psychological state of belief is correctly ascribed both by the quasi-reduction and by the means we employ when there is no expression in a person's language of his beliefs. What makes both states *belief*? The fundamental problem, once again, for the defender of the quasi-reduction is that if he attempts to answer this question by pointing to some common role that belief plays in both cases – for instance its satisfaction of the *a priori* principles and the intertemporal constraints upon its application – then this role is something we can use in the case of a language-using creature to circumvent the radical interpretation procedure. If the role is properly specified in the answer to the question raised by the objector then a state identified as fulfilling that role will be

[26] The quasi-reduction does indeed tie holding-true to other concepts, for instance that of saying. But it is not plausible to suppose that these other concepts could be possessed by someone who does not know what it is to have a particular belief.

[27] On the matter of the attribution of attitudes to languageless creatures, I am in agreement with Jonathan Bennett in *Linguistic Behaviour* (Cambridge: CUP, 1976) and D. Armstrong in *Belief, Truth and Knowledge* (Cambridge: CUP 1973); but for some disagreements with Bennett over Davidson's radical interpretation procedure, see my review of his book in the *Journal of Philosophy* 74 (1977) at 368–9.

belief; if it is not belief, then the question was not properly answered in the first place.

It may be protested that this is too hasty. Perhaps the role given in answer to the question is not sufficiently rich to determine what someone believes, although it is not inadequate as an answer to the question of what makes all these states differently identified beliefs. Now there are two different things that may be meant here by 'not sufficiently rich'. One is that the role given would not be sufficient to fix the contents of belief for a language-using creature even to the limited extent to which we do in fact hold them to be determinate. But then the force of the original objection is not really answered: for the extra that does determine the contents for nonlinguistic creatures has not been shown to be unified with the determination of the detailed beliefs of a language-using person via the radical interpretation procedure. On the other hand 'not sufficiently rich' may mean that while belief has a common role in all the kinds of case so far cited, there will be extra constraints to which it is subject when a person has a language, and in particular there will be links with the concept of *saying that* and *assertion*. But this still does not show that the quasi-reduction's method cannot be circumvented: for we could identify several alternative sets of beliefs for an agent with a language, by whatever was given as the common role of belief, and then eliminate some of these sets by further restrictions relating to saying and assertion, if there really are additional constraints in the linguistic case.[28] The correct conclusion in all these cases seems to be that what shows a quasi-reduction to be a quasi-reduction precisely for the notion for which it purports to be, also shows that the quasi-reduction is unnecessary.

(3) The third classification under which an alleged quasi-reduction which employs holding-true as its concept Q may fall, is specified by dropping the requirement of case (2) that the attitudes employed in identifying holding-true be identifiable in advance of interpretation of the sentences which were to be interpreted by the quasi-reduction. The word 'alleged' is

---

[28] In fact it seems more plausible to say not that there are additional *constraints*, but that in the linguistic case the evidential base for the identification of psychological states that satisfy given, common constraints is much *richer* than in the nonlinguistic case.

present here because it is clear that the difficulty for such a view is going to lie in the defence of the claim that we still have in this case a genuine quasi-reduction. The picture to be offered by a theory falling under this case is presumably that the detailed attitudes and interpretations are ascribed *en bloc*, any links between belief, desire, holding-true, and meaning now functioning as constraints on the legitimacy of applying the whole package. Naturally it is no part of my aim to object to this conception as such, for it is close to the view that I wish to defend: the question now is only whether any distinctive quasi-reductive role is still being played on this view by the concept of holding-true. I deny that it is.

Under the view in question, there seems to be no special status relevant to the possibility of a quasi-reduction, which is enjoyed by holding-true and not enjoyed by detailed ascriptions of attitudes and meanings. In the case both of such detailed ascriptions and of holding-true, temporarily taking the remainder of the semantical and psychological truths about the person and his sentences as fixed, we can check that a given claim about holding-true or about detailed attitudes or meanings has the consequences in the agent's behaviour we would expect; and we can check that no simpler or more sophisticated attribution is respectively sufficient or necessary in the circumstances, taking into account what the agent does on all other occasions. Similarly on this view we cannot attribute any one of the trio of detailed attitudes, holding-true, or meanings, in advance of the remaining two. If holding-true is playing a 'central role'[29] in interpretation here, it is a role also played by the detailed ascriptions too. There of course remains a sense in which holding (and wishing, etc.) true fails to have entailments to detailed ascriptions of attitude: but this is just failure to make assumptions in the sense (1) we distinguished earlier, and saw to be no help to the radical interpreter following Davidson's procedure.

Before continuing the discussion of possible quasi-reductions, I should make a disclaimer. I have been arguing against the possibility of holding-true playing the role of the concept Q of a quasi-reduction of (some fragment of) the action explanation scheme: I do not mean to imply that holding-true does not

---

[29] 'Thought and Talk', p. 14.

have *some* role to play in a radical interpretation procedure that is not a quasi-reduction. Certainly we must recognize that there is no reason why there must be a uniform, projectible behavioural manifestation – disjunctive definitions included – of holding-true, even for a given person, let alone a community: for holding-true is defined in terms of belief, and we have seen that there are no particular behavioural manifestations of *that*. Nevertheless, one can still make initial, revisable guesses about who holds which sentences true; indeed (as John McDowell has remarked) a procedure – Davidson's or some other – which suggests a hypothesis about the entire meaning theory from such guesses supplies something that guesses about detailed beliefs expressed in utterances on particular occasions cannot by themselves supply – a set of interlocking hypotheses about the sense of many sentences simultaneously. My point is just that one can be as reasonably convinced of a particular belief that someone is expressing it, or can be as convinced of the subject matter of that person's belief (e.g. his biological needs) as one is of a claim about holding-true; reasonable provisional guesses about such detailed beliefs should equally constrain selection of a hypothesis about the meaning theory. Holding-true has an important role, but it is not evidentially prior to these other sources of evidence.[30]

4. INTEGRATED QUASI-REDUCTIONS

The more general conclusion to be drawn from these arguments about holding-true is not (or not yet, anyway) that a quasi-reduction cannot be given; for someone attracted to the possibility of supplying such a quasi-reduction for the scheme of holistic explanation of action may justly reply that while the objections just given do apply against a quasi-reduction taking holding-true as its concept Q, this may only be because we have not yet dug deep enough. What we need to consider, it will be said, is the possibility of a quasi-reduction yielding as output simultaneously beliefs, desires and sentence-senses, a quasi-reduction that does not presuppose the availability of any one

---

[30] I do not mean to imply by my omission of them that there are not other major difficulties with Davidson's radical interpretation procedure: my concern has been with the concept Q he chose rather than the method M, or his claim that his method will filter out non-interpretational truth theories.

of these in advance of a construction of a theory of the remainder of them. The plausibility of the demand for a quasi-reduction in the action case will have to rest on the possibility of such an *integrated* quasi-reduction; for that is where the weight of any such requirement must fall. If our arguments so far are correct, then from the point of view of someone requiring a quasi-reduction, as Davidson seems to, the possibility of such an integrated theory is not, as Davidson sometimes seems to suggest in his writings, the possibility of there existing a true, happily unified theory on the chances of which one may 'speculate',[31] but a necessary condition of the scheme of holistic explanation having empirical application at all. Thus we need to consider in some detail the prospects for such an integrated quasi-reduction.

We may schematically represent Davidson's radical interpretation procedure and Ramsey's decision theory respectively by the upper and lower forked arrows below: the concepts at the tails of each arrow are those such that truths stated using them have as a resultant truths stated using the concept at the

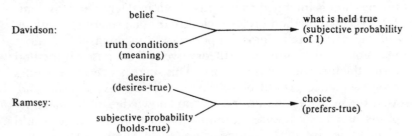

head of the arrow. Pursuing the metaphor we may say that each method gives an account of how truths about what is held true or what is chosen may be resolved into the component forces from which they result. This representation suggests one, and what is perhaps the only, plausible way of integrating the two theories. If we construe the concepts on the lower arrow as attitudes to sentences, then it is clear that what is at the head of the upper arrow is a special case of what is at the lower fork of the lower arrow: for a sentence to be held true is for it to have a high degree of subjective probability. So the natural integrated procedure is that determined by the diagram when

[31] 'Belief and the Basis of Meaning', p. 316.

the upper arrow is repositioned so that its output is the input of the lower fork of Ramsey's arrow. Thus in such an integrated theory, the fundamental concept in the quasi-reduction will be that of preferring true (at a given time) one sentence to another, where it is essential to the method that these sentences may be complex.

The first stage of such a procedure would consist in the application of a decision theory to the preference ordering of sentences in order to obtain subjective probabilities and desirabilities. I have referred to Ramsey, but in fact Richard Jeffrey has offered convincing reasons for not making use, as Ramsey does, of the causal notion of a gamble:[32] for any sentence *s* on which there is *some* gamble in the preference ordering (and there must be some such *s* for Ramsey's method to be applicable), for Ramsey the preference ordering must contain gambles on *s* with respect to *any* other two sentences in the ordering. Consideration of some such gambles ('A revolution next week if the coin lands heads, a wet summer otherwise') as genuinely possible will make the subject revise the beliefs that the method is intended to identify, both in degree and content. Jeffrey's own method involves closure of the preference ranking only under certain logical operators, and to assess a more plausible kind of integrated theory, we will suppose his method forms the first stage of the theory. This stage, since the attitudes are to sentences, could be carried out by an investigator who, as at the next stage too, as yet has no knowledge of the meaning of his subject's sentences. Completion of this first stage would yield subjective probabilities of sentences to which Davidson's method, using the Principle of Charity qualified by causal and epistemological constraints, is then applied in the second stage to yield truth conditions and thereby beliefs. Davidson has always insisted that all kinds of epistemological theories may enter the assessment of a proposed interpretation of the subject's tongue, and the fact that the first stage of the procedure yields detailed degrees of belief only increases the richness of the evidential base made available to the second stage.

This is an impressive and indeed arresting construction, but can it really be made to serve the purposes of a quasi-reduction? Doubts are produced by the use as fundamental of the concept

[32] *The Logic of Decision* (New York: McGraw-Hill, 1965), pp. 146 ff.

of preferring-true: we need access to truths about such preferences for the procedure to be applicable. Preferences as
expressed in behaviour yield actions, that is, token events: and
these token events, being each one an instance of ever so many
types, in advance of a theory of interpretation give no clue to
the *type* (or indeed *believed* type) for which the behaviour
expresses preference; nor do they give any connection with a
particular sentence of the subject's language. We need rather
something that stands to the two-place relation (*modulo* agent
and time reference) of preferring-true, as Quine's procedure of
query and assent stands to the one-place concept of holding-
true.

Someone might suggest we could meet that need as follows.
We may present two sentences of his language to our subject,
the presenter may then make a response to first one of them,
and then make true the one to which he has responded: then
it may be hoped that the subject will catch on to the idea that
if *he* responds, the sentence thus picked out will come true. But
it should be obvious that this suggestion is utterly vacuous,
since the whole procedure was meant to yield *inter alia* the truth
conditions of the subject's sentences, whereas under this
proposal these would already have to be known to the investigator in order for him to know how to make true (if he could
at all) a sentence of the subject's language. So even Ramsey's
antecedent in this sentence he wrote is not sufficient:

If then we had the power of the Almighty, and could persuade our
subject of our power, we could, by offering him options, discover
how he placed in order of merit all possible courses of the world.[33]

(Omnipotence is not enough. We would also need some part of
the Almighty's omniscience about our subject.) I have not
myself been able to see how this difficulty could be overcome.

There are of course other complications. The first stage of the
procedure requires that we be able to identify some truth-
functional connectives in the subject's language. This, it may
be said, can easily be done, using the facts about any signs for
conjunction, negation, and so forth summarized in what Quine
calls their respective verdict tables. But quite apart from the
possible absence of any such connectives in his language, there

---

[33] 'Truth and Probability' in *The Foundations of Mathematics*, p. 176.

is the familiar point, granted by Quine himself,[34] that a putative sign of assent may be rejected as such if it produces 'extra-ordinary difficulties', among which, we may add, will be the failure of the held-true sentences (in the sense in which 'holding-true' is a sign of assent) to generate a set of beliefs that meet all the other constraints (causal constraints, a constraint that they be explanatory of action, etc.) we wish to place upon them. It might be suggested that we should pick on a sign of assent only after completion of the first stage of the integrated procedure, so that we could check it against what is held true. But this is again an incoherent proposal, for we needed a sign of assent to identify the connectives which we in turn needed to carry out the initial half of the procedure in the first place.

Nothing we have said here constitutes in any sense a *proof* that a quasi-reduction cannot be given for this scheme of holistic explanation.[35] Nevertheless the failures in each particular proposal are connected; and we have seen in another case, the spatial case, how a quasi-reduction is in no way a prerequisite for application of the scheme. For these reasons it seems dogmatic always to require a quasi-reduction for a system of holistic explanation. If one wanted a slogan to express the view which all these arguments encourage, one might do worse than this: the verification of the applicability of a scheme of holistic explanation is itself holistic.

[34] *Words and Objections* (Dordrecht: Reidel, 1970), eds. D. Davidson and J. Hintikka, p. 312.

[35] I have, for instance, ignored evidence that might be said to be available for a quasi-reduction from ψ-ing-true for other propositional attitudes verbs as substituends for 'ψ'. (For such a resource to be of any use here, one would of course need a procedure related to these attitudes as Davidson's alleged radical interpretation procedure stands to the attitude of holding-true: the availability of such a procedure seems to be an open question.) But analogous arguments to that given for holding-true apply to any one of these attitudes. We may fix, for instance, upon that of fearing-true: it is clear that there is no one action-type whose instances are identifiable in advance of attribution of detailed propositional attitudes which shows that a subject fears a certain sentence to be true. This observation remains true even if there were a linguistic mood of sentences that stood to fear as the indicative actually stands to belief: for nothing can prevent the (intentionally or unintentionally) misleading use of a sentence of no matter what conceivable mood.

INDEX*

A posteriori principles, 162-4, 169
A priori principles, 27-30, 39, 54
  as partly distinctive of holistic explanation, 21-2
  for action, 11
  for perception, 16
Absolute space—*see* space
Action:
  akratic, 31-2
  and physical events, 116-7
  causal theory of, 56, 171
  irrational—*see* akratic
  'vestibule of', 94n.
Anscombe, G. E. M., 169-71
Armstrong, D., 209n.
Ayer, A. J., 3-6, 11, 12n.

B-state, 114-5
B-truth, 18-9, 33, 37
Behaviourism:
  definitional, 20
  logical, 119
Belief:
  irrational, 32
  irreducibility principle for—*see* Irreducibility principle
  physical definition of, 23-4
Benaceraff, P., 81n.
Bennett, J., 8-10, 186n., 209n.
Boyd, R., 41n.
Brain states:
  as explanatory of action, 6n.
  and mastery of E-concepts, 23
Bratman, M., 32
Burge, T., 175
Butler, R. J., 74n.

Causal theories:
  of perception, 56
  of rational action—*see* Action
Charity, principle of, 202n., 214
Clarke, S., 44
Collingwood, R. G., 154
Conjunction restriction, 147-53, 161-4
Contingency, illusion of—*see* Kripke
Counterfactual theories:
  of causation, 76, 167n.
  of nondeviance in causal chains, 75-9
Counterfactuals:
  in defining deviant causal chains, 56-7, 75-6
  sustained by covering laws, 78
  sustained in counterfactual theories of nondeviance, 78-9

Davidson, D., 14n., 19-20, 36n., 40, 66, 111-3, 135-6, 155n., 171n., 179-80, 196-216
Dennett, D., 119n.
Desires:
  as 'pro attitudes', 14n.
  as reasons for acting, 14
  physical definition of, 23-4
Dispositions:
  'many track', 4, 149, 152
  to form beliefs, 32
Duhem, -'s thesis, 35-6
Dummett, M., 19, 44n.

E-concepts, 18, 20-1, 29, 31-2, 34-5, 37-8, 54, 109, 124, 165, 179, 181, 190, 192
  basis for the application of, 22-5, 27-8, 113
  mastery of, 21-2, 28, 35
E-state, 114-5
E-truth, 18, 20, 31, 55, 109, 181, 184
Earman, J., 42
Epiphenomenalism, 119
Essentialism:
  about states, 60
Evans, G., 44n., 45, 143n.
Experience:
  and the concept of an objective world, 184
  'as of' a certain kind, 18n.
Explanation:
  and 'because', 171
  Hempelian (deductive-nomological), 160-1
  qualitative, 127-31
  reference fixing, 127-31
  restriction on covering law model, 12-3
  strong differential, 79-80

Feature-placing vocabulary, 46-8
Field, H., 53n., 173-4
Functionalism, 117
Functions:
  specified in laws invoked in explanation, 66-7

Goldman, A. I., 71n., 105n.
Grandy, R., 37-8
Grice, H. P., 37-8, 39-40, 77n., 88n., 95, 101n., 156, 203

Harman, G., 15n., 83-4, 88n.
Hellman, G., 122n.

* I am grateful to Teresa Rosen for her assistance in the preparation of this index.

Holding-true, 179, 181, 196–216
Holism:
   holistically connected components, 34
   in explanation, 18–9
   in respect of the evidence, 19
   intertemporal constraints, 30–5, 37, 190–1
Hornsby, J., 66n.
Hume, D., 14

Identity thesis:
   state-state, 119
   token-token, 116n., 132, 134–5
   type-type, 117, 125–6, 131, 133, 139
Imagination:
   perceptual, 131n.
   sympathetic, 131n.
Independent verifiability, requirement of, 145–6
Indexical reference, 175–8
Intentionality, 11
   as relational, 73–4
Intentions:
   as causes of behavior, 12n.
   as required in a priori principles, 15
   irreducibility to desire and belief, 15–6
Irreducibility:
   of indexical reference, 175
   to behavior, 17–8
   to intention, 17–8
   semantic, 172–4
Irreducibility principle:
   for belief to action-types, 5
   for desire to action-types, 5
   for location to experience-kinds, 7
   for properties of places to experience-kinds, 7–8

Jeffrey, R., 214

Kaplan, D., 12n., 130, 143n.
Kenny, A., 56
Kinglake, -'s hallucination, 75n.
Knowledge:
   causal theory of, 25
Kripke, S., 81n., 124–34, 143n.

Laws:
   connecting behavior, 4
   connecting perceptual experiences, 6
   covering, 68, 70, 78, 145–6, 147
   in differential explanation, 66
   in schemes of holistic explanation, 69n.
   psychophysical, 153–4

Leibniz, G. W. von, 44
Leibniz, -'s law, 142n.
Lewis, D., 78, 118n., 135, 139–43, 173–4

Mackie, J. L., 67–8
Malcolm, N., 119
McDowell, J., 16n., 166n., 212
McGinn, C., 133n.
Meaning:
   given in terms of criteria, 25
Morton, A., 57–8

Nagel, T., 14, 118, 131n., 172–8
Necessity:
   epistemic, 10–11
   metaphysical, 10–11
No-explanation view, 153–65
Non-subsumption view, 153, 154–5

O'Shaughnessy, B., 90n.

Pears, D., 86, 88–95, 98n., 101n., 170
Physical Embedding, Principle of, 123–4
Piaget, J., 188, 194
Places:
   identity conditions of, 49–52
   pre-, 182–9, 193
   properties of, 3
Poincaré, H., 194–5
Preference ordering—see Ramsey, F. P.
Preferring-true, 215
Price, H. H., 77n.
Principles:
   a priori—see A priori principles
   a posteriori—see A posteriori principles
   invoked in explanation, 66–7
Psychological feudalism, 89
Putnam, H., 23n., 41n., 116, 128, 143

Quasi-functional statements:
   about objects, 28
Quasi-reduction—see Reduction
Quine, W. V., 8n., 22n., 45, 83n., 215–6

Railton, P., 166n.
Ramsey, F. P., 180, 213–5
Rationality, 31–3, 190–1
Realization:
   in causal contexts, 117–22
   of psychological states, 69–70, 116, 121, 144
Recoverability, condition of:
   jump, 79–81
   stepwise, 80–4
Reducibility—see Irreducibility

Reduction:
  higher-order physical definition, 23–4
  of action to belief-desire pairs, 5–6
  of perception, 6
  of spatial concepts, 8–10
  nomological, 172–4
  non-qualitative, 47–54
  quasi-, 179–81, 194–5, 207–11, 212–16
Reliability, 91–2
Ryle, G., 4

Sacks, O., 87n.
Schiffer, S., 39
Sensitivity, 57, 59, 61, 63, 69, 74, 79
Sklar, L., 42n., 44n., 45n.
Sosa, E., 152n.
Space,
  absolute, 10, 41
  absoluteness$_1$, 42, 44–5
  absoluteness$_2$, 43
  location in—see location
  pre-, 182–9, 193

Specific reflection, 69
Strawson, P. F., 8, 44n., 75, 86, 95–9, 101n., 182n.
Supervenience:
  of a psychological state on a physical
    state, 48, 70n., 121

Taylor, C., 12n., 24, 151n.
Thalberg, I., 57n.
Thompson, F., 122n.
Transitivity:
  converse of (for 'differentially explains'), 68–9, 71
  of 'differentially explains', 68

Unger, P., 134n.

von Wright, G. H., 154
Wiggins, D., 143n.
Wittgenstein, L., 199n.